THE
ANTI-AGEING
BIBLE

By the same author from Souvenir Press

THE FOOD MEDICINE BIBLE

THE
ANTI-AGEING
BIBLE

*Nature's Secret Weapons Against the
Ageing Process*

Earl Mindell, R.Ph., Ph.D.

SOUVENIR PRESS

Copyright © 1995 by Earl Mindell, R.Ph., Ph.D., and Carol Colman

The right of Earl Mindell to be identified as author of
this work has been asserted by him in accordance with
the Copyright, Designs and Patents Act 1988.

First published in the U.S.A. as a
Fireside Book by Simon & Schuster, New York,
under the title *Earl Mindell's Anti-Aging Bible*

First British edition published 1995 by
Souvenir Press Ltd,
43 Great Russell Street, London WC1B 3PA

Reprinted 2000

ISBN 0 285 63274 4

Photoset by Rowland Phototypesetting Ltd
Bury St Edmunds, Suffolk

Printed in Great Britain by
The Guernsey Press Co. Ltd, Guernsey, Channel Islands

Contents

Chapter 1

Maximum Maintenance: Maximum Health

Of all the spectacular advances in medicine, science and technology that have occurred over the past hundred years the ones that have had the most profound impact on our lives are those that have increased the human life span. In 1900 the average life expectancy for people in the developed nations was 47 years. Today, as we approach the dawn of a new century, the average life span has increased by more than 50 per cent to 76 years. The fastest growing segment of the population consists of men and women aged 75 and older, a group referred to by gerontologists as the 'old old'. The number of octogenarians among us continues to grow, and some scientists say that a life span of about 115 years may eventually be the norm. Others contend that biological engineering will extend our life span to 150 years, and a few insist that humans could one day live to be as old as 400!

The increase in life span that we have experienced during this century is primarily due to improved sanitation, the elimination of many lethal childhood diseases through vaccination, and other medical advances such as the development of antibiotics. Although rare today, death from infection during childbirth was a leading cause of mortality among women at the turn of the century. Thanks to penicillin and its 'wonder drug' offspring, bacterial infections such as pneumonia and streptococcus are no longer life-threatening. Although heart disease is still the leading cause of death in the West, the resulting mortality rate is declining due to better prevention and more aggressive treatments. Cancer continues to be the second most common cause of death, but the prognosis for at least certain forms of the disease has vastly improved within the past century. We owe a debt of gratitude to the scientists and doctors who have brought us this far, but there are limits to what they have been able to do. Members of the medical establishment readily acknowledge that although we have managed to extend the length of life, in many cases we have done little to improve its quality. A recent editorial in a medical magazine lamented the fact that 'the ratio of active life to disabled or functionally compromised life has not increased and may actually have diminished during the last quarter of a century.' (*Patient Care*, 28 February, 1994.) In other words, people may be living longer, but they're not living better.

Despite the increase in life span, the perception of ageing as a depressing downward spiral of growing wrinkled, growing senile, growing ill and growing old persists. Indeed, for many of today's elderly people, growing older is synonymous with increasing ill health. Nearly half of all people over 65 are taking some form of medication and their lives are punctuated by visits to the doctor and the hospital. In addition to life-threatening diseases, life-diminishing diseases such as arthritis, vision problems, memory loss and sleep disorders continue to plague the elderly.

This does not have to be the case. Sadly, and ironically, too many people suffer from ailments that are easily preventable or controllable through diet and lifestyle. According to the American National Cancer Institute, as many as 35 per cent of all cancers may be due to poor diet. Experts estimate that at least 50 per cent of all cases of heart disease might be averted by changes in diet and lifestyle which in themselves would greatly enhance both the length and quality of life.

Why and how we age is still very much a mystery. Serious research on ageing is relatively new and only a few scientists are doing concentrated work in this area. Until recently, many were disdainful of colleagues involved in ageing research, likening it to alchemy or the pursuit of the mythical fountain of youth. However, as the population has begun to age, interest in the ageing process and age-related illnesses has begun to attract greater attention.

In the past there was a fatalistic attitude towards ageing that was shared by both experts and lay persons alike; they believed that there was little they could do to prevent the 'ravages' of growing old. Today, we know better: there is strong evidence that the downward spiral is not inevitable. For one thing, although they are still in the minority, there is a growing population of 'old old' people who are ageing well and who have managed to stay active and healthy. We see them on tennis courts, in adult education classes, in the gym and sometimes still in active employment. Researchers have begun to study the lives and lifestyles of these successful agers, in the hope of discovering important information that will help us all age well. Throughout the world they are finding new and exciting ways to maintain health and vitality well into old age, and innovative techniques to prevent some of the common ailments associated with ageing. Scientists all over the United States are engaged in research that has generated important information on why and how we age. Here are some of their fascinating findings:

- Vitamins and supplements (antioxidants) may help to protect the body against compounds that are thought to speed up the ageing process.
- A handful of foods and supplements may substantially reduce the risk of developing cataracts and macular degeneration, the leading cause of blindness among the elderly.
- An ancient herb and other supplements may help to prevent memory loss and keep your mind alert and sharp.
- Vitamins and supplements may help to rejuvenate a 'tired' immune system.
- Contrary to the popular belief that our muscles grow weaker as we age, it is actually possible, with the right kind of exercise, to build muscle and maintain strength well into our nineties and beyond.
- A supplement widely used in Japan as a treatment for heart disease (and available at health food shops) may help to keep an ageing heart pumping as strongly as a younger one.
- Prostate problems (common among men over 50) may be

prevented or reversed by a combination of diet and supplements.
- The right combination of herbs and supplements can relieve the discomfort of menopause for many women.

Here is more good news: these tools are readily available to anyone who wants to use them. For the first time we have the power and the knowledge to change our fate and make a real difference in both the quality and the length of our lives. Although the sooner we start the better, positive changes can produce positive results at any stage of life.

This book will show you how to get started. In *The Anti-Ageing Bible* I examine the latest research on ageing and show how you can use this information to help you live a longer, healthier life. I have compiled a list of the 'Hot Hundred' anti-ageing substances—foods, vitamins, supplements, herbs and other compounds—that can help you age successfully. With few exceptions, they are easily obtainable from chemists, grocers and health food shops. I devote special, separate chapters to the unique ageing issues that confront men and women, and perhaps most importantly, in the chapter 'Staying Well: A Guide to Preventing the Common Ailments of Ageing', I stress prevention and drug-free approaches to dealing with many problems that can seriously interfere with the quality of our lives.

Finally, I want to stress that the techniques I describe in this book are not a fountain of youth, although they can help us retain our youthfulness. An 80-year-old who follows my suggestions is not going to look or feel the same as a 20-year-old. What I am suggesting is that an 80-year-old can be vigorous, strong, attractive and full of life. My goal is not to turn back the clock, but to help you be the best 50-, 60-, 70-, 80- or even 100-year-old you can be.

Chapter 2

The 'Hot Hundred'
Anti-Ageing Arsenal
from A to Z

The anti-ageing 'Hot Hundred' contains a select group of vitamins, minerals, foods, herbs and other supplements that can help us live longer, healthier lives. Except for the rare drug or supplement that may be available on prescription only, the anti-ageing 'Hot Hundred' are available at health food shops, chemists, herbalists and, in some cases, at your local supermarket.

CAUTION   If you are taking a prescription drug for a medical condition, do not discontinue the drug without first consulting your doctor or natural healer.

ACIDOPHILUS

FACTS   Several years ago, an American television commercial for a popular brand of yogurt contended that eating yogurt was the key to longevity. The commercial featured several centenarians from an obscure part of rural Russia who had one thing in common: they were all lifelong yogurt eaters. At the time, the premise of the commercial may have sounded a bit far-fetched, but scientists are now discovering that there might be something in it after all.

11

Yogurt contains *Lactobacillus acidophilus* (commonly known as acidophilus) a so-called 'friendly bacterium' that is used to ferment milk into yogurt, and is also present in the gastrointestinal tract. Acidophilus not only aids digestion, but appears to help keep in check the growth of yeast, such as *Candida albicans*, which is the cause of many vaginal yeast infections. In fact, acidophilus is a common folk remedy for yeast infection, but more importantly, recent studies suggest that acidophilus may help the body ward off other infections as well.

Acidophilus is present in yogurt and is also available in tablets or powder form.

THE RIGHT AMOUNT   Eat two 250 g cartons of low fat yogurt with active cultures daily. (Be sure the carton specifies *active cultures*.)

Take two acidophilus tablets three times daily, half an hour before or after meals.

Mix one packet of acidophilus powder in 150 ml of freshly squeezed juice, one or two times daily.

POSSIBLE BENEFITS

Anti-fungal. Women who are menopausal should take note: the vaginal dryness that often accompanies the drop in oestrogen can make you more prone to vaginal yeast infections. A carton or two of yogurt a day may be just what the doctor ordered.

Those are the findings of a woman doctor at Long Island Jewish Medical Center, who recently studied the effectiveness of acidophilus against vaginal yeast infections. In her study she instructed women with a history of chronic yeast infection to eat 250 g of yogurt (with live acidophilus cultures) each day and compared them to non-yogurt eaters. After six months, the women who ate the yogurt had far fewer yeast infections than those who did not.

Immune Booster. As we age our immune systems weaken, making us more vulnerable to infections of all kinds. A carton of yogurt a day may help to maintain normal immune function. A researcher at the University of California studied the effects of yogurt with live cultures on the immune system. His findings: people who ate two 250 g cartons of yogurt daily had higher blood levels of gamma-interferon, a substance that helps the body to ward off infection. He also noticed that the people who ate yogurt with live cultures also had substantially fewer colds and allergy symptoms than those who did not.

PERSONAL ADVICE   I am frequently asked whether acidophilus capsules are as good as eating yogurt with live cultures. Actually, the capsules and granules provide a more potent form of acidophilus. Sometimes the capsules or granules are preferable, especially if you have a yeast problem or are taking an antibiotic that is wreaking havoc with your digestive system by killing off the friendly bacteria. (Erythromycin is a particular offender.) However, under normal circumstances, eating yogurt is probably good enough. In addition, yogurt offers the added benefit of a hefty boost of calcium, which is needed for strong bones and normal blood pressure and heart function.

ALLIUM VEGETABLES

FACTS   There are 500 plants belonging to the genus *Allium*, including garlic, onion, chives, shallots and other related vegetables. The American National Cancer Society is investigating many members of the allium family for their potential cancer-fighting properties. In addition, researchers have found that these special vegetables may be helpful in the prevention and treatment of a wide range of ailments including Alzheimer's disease and cardiovascular disease, two problems that are particularly prevalent among the older population.

THE RIGHT AMOUNT   Use these vegetables liberally in your cooking! Red and yellow onions and shallots have the highest flavonoid content of allium vegetables. (Flavonoids may protect against cancer.)

Fresh garlic should be eaten daily—I prefer to bake or stir-fry it; it has a milder flavour than eating it raw. If you can't stomach the stuff, try using odourless garlic capsules. Take one or two capsules after each meal daily. Try taking them with an internal breath freshener made from parsley seed oil or chlorella.

POSSIBLE BENEFITS

Alzheimer's Disease. At a 1994 meeting on medicinal foods organised by Rutger's University, French researchers reported on a study involving aged laboratory rats with an Alzheimer's type disease. The researchers noted that garlic extract appeared to slow down brain deterioration. In addition, the garlic normalised the brain's serotonin system—if the serotonin system malfunctions, it can cause depression. Although this information is exciting, it is not yet known whether garlic would have the same effect on human brains.

Cancer Fighter. Hippocrates, the father of modern medicine, used garlic vapours to treat uterine cancer. Recent studies have shown that people who eat a diet high in allium vegetables, including garlic, have a lower rate of stomach cancer than those who do not. Researchers in China interviewed 564 patients with stomach cancer and more than 1,100 people without cancer in a region where the risk for gastric cancer is high. Those with the highest intake of allium vegetables had a 40 per cent reduction in risk for gastric cancer.

Garlic and onion are both rich in quercetin and selenium, two 'hot' antioxidants that may play an important role in cancer prevention.

Garlic oil contains diallyl sulphide which has been shown to deactivate potent carcinogens in animal studies. Garlic also stimulates the production of glutathione, a potent antioxidant found in the cells that help to prevent cancerous changes.

Heart Disease. The first-century physician Dioscorides prescribed garlic to treat atherosclerosis, a leading cause of heart disease. Indeed, numerous studies can attest to garlic's positive effects on blood lipids. In a recent study performed at the Clinical Research Center and Tulane University School of Medicine in New Orleans, 42 healthy adults with total cholesterol levels over 200 mg/dl were given either 300 mg of standardised garlic powder in tablet form three times daily or a placebo. After 12 weeks, those who took the garlic experienced a six per cent total drop in cholesterol versus a one per cent decline among those on the placebo. Even better, those on the garlic had an 11 per cent reduction in LDL or 'bad' cholesterol against a three per cent drop in the untreated group.

Other studies have shown that people who eat an onion a day can raise their HDL or 'good' cholesterol.

Researcher Eric Block discovered a compound in garlic called ajoene that appears to be a natural blood thinner, which may prevent the formation of blood clots that can lead to a heart attack or stroke.

Natural Antibiotic, Anti-fungal. In the Middle Ages, monks used garlic to ward off plague. Before antibiotics, garlic poultices were used on wounds to prevent infection. In fact, garlic was dubbed 'Russian penicillin' because during World War II when antibiotics were scarce, Russian doctors used it to treat infections on the battlefield. Studies show that garlic has some antibiotic properties and is also one of the strongest natural anti-fungal compounds, especially against *Candida albicans* (yeast infection).

Anti-inflammatory. Eric Block recently discovered a sulphur compound in onion which, in test tube studies, blocked the chemical chain of events that lead to asthma and inflammatory reactions.

Only nine per cent of all UK citizens eat six or more fruits and vegetables daily as recommended by the Department of Health. According to experts, as many as fifty per cent of all cancers could be prevented by eating the right foods.

ALOE

FACTS   There are more than 300 species of the aloe plant, and several, including the famous aloe vera variety, have been used since ancient times to heal skin wounds. Aloe gel, derived from the leaf of the plant, is an excellent moisturiser and is a common ingredient in skin creams. Several studies confirm that, used externally, aloe can promote healing of minor skin burns and abrasions. Recently, a study performed on animals at Texas A&M University showed that, taken internally, aloe may be a potent immune booster.

THE RIGHT AMOUNT   Aloe gel may be used liberally on the skin as needed. The leaf of the fresh plant is highly effective, but if you don't want to grow your own, aloe vera is available in many different forms at chemists' shops and health food shops. Buy only products that are made from pure aloe and that list aloe as a primary ingredient. Many products that claim to contain aloe contain a watered down version of aloe extract or reconstituted aloe vera. Aloe, which is used as a treatment for constipation, can cause severe abdominal pain and cramps if taken in large amounts. One tablespoon (10 ml) one to two times daily is recommended. Aloe vera is also available in dry capsule form. Each capsule is equal to one tablespoon (10 ml) of the juice.

CAUTION   Aloe in capsule form should not be used by pregnant women.

POSSIBLE BENEFITS

Wound Healing. Several studies have shown that aloe vera gel can help heal skin irritations and wounds due to radiation burns. At one time, researchers believed that aloe vera promoted healing by sealing in moisture, thus preventing the air from drying out the skin. However, scientists now suspect that there are specific chemicals in aloe vera gel which interact with the skin to speed up the healing process.

Wrinkles. Like other moisturisers, aloe gel may give the appearance of younger-looking skin by plumping out dry, fine lines. Thus, the wrinkles don't disappear, but they are less noticeable.

Immune Booster. This is one of the newest and most exciting uses of this ancient herb. Researchers at Texas A&M University tested aloe on mice implanted with sarcoma tumours. Mice who had been given aloe vera internally had a 40 per cent survival rate. All of the untreated mice died. Interestingly enough, researchers found that it was impossible to implant tumours in mice who had been pretreated with aloe vera. Researchers say that the compound works by stimulating the release of cytokines, substances which activate the immune system. Aloe is now being tested on human patients.

ALPHA-CAROTENE

FACTS The carotene family consists of about 600 naturally occurring compounds found in dark, leafy vegetables and yellow and orange fruits and vegetables. Some of these compounds are potent antioxidants, such as beta-carotene and lycopene. However, only a handful of carotenes have actually been studied for their potential health benefits. Recently, researchers have focused on alpha-carotene and their findings suggest that it may be as important a cancer fighter as any of its better known cousins.

THE RIGHT AMOUNT There is no RDA for alpha-carotene. Fruits and vegetables are a rich source of many different carotenes, including alpha-carotenes. For example, about one-third of the carotene mixture in a carrot consists of alpha-carotene. Supplements containing alpha- and beta-carotene are available at health food shops. Take between 10,000 and 25,000 iu daily.

POSSIBLE BENEFITS
Cancer Fighter. For more than a decade, studies have shown that people whose diets are rich in green and yellow vegetables have significantly lower rates of cancer than those who eat little or none of these. Many scientists believe that carotenes are responsible for the reduced cancer risk.

A recent study compared the effect of alpha- and beta-carotene, and of no carotene, on cancer cells in a culture medium. High levels of alpha-carotene stopped the growth of the cancer cells. An equal amount of beta-carotene produced a modest drop in cell growth. However, the cancer cells without any form of carotene experienced explosive growth.

17

In another study, reported in the journal *Cancer Research*, mice were fed a known carcinogen and then divided into three groups. One group of the mice was fed a beta-carotene supplement, a second group was given an alpha-carotene supplement and the third group was given a placebo. The mice taking the alpha-carotene had a 70 per cent reduction in the number of tumours as against those taking the beta-carotene or no supplement at all. From these studies, researchers suspect that alpha-carotene may be a better protector against certain forms of cancer than beta-carotene.

PERSONAL ADVICE   I recommend taking a caretenoid complex along with dark green leafy vegetables, and yellow and orange vegetables and fruits. It comes in liquid, tablet or capsule form. Use as directed.

ALPHA-HYDROXY ACIDS

FACTS   Alpha-hydroxy acids (AHA) are naturally occurring compounds found in foods such as sour milk (lactic acid), grapes (tartaric acid), sugar cane (glycolic acid), apples (malic acid) and citrus fruit (citric acid). For more than a decade, dermatologists have used high concentrations of alpha-hydroxy acids (up to 50 per cent) for scar removal and facial peels. Today, weaker versions of AHA are sold in numerous over-the-counter skin care produces designed to moisturise and improve the skin. Although they may not be the fountain of youth, for many people, AHA products can produce noticeable changes in the appearance and quality of their skin.

THE RIGHT AMOUNT   Products range from two to ten per cent concentration of AHA. Most dermatologists consider five per cent or under to be safe for most people. However, some people may find AHA irritating at any level, and some may be able to tolerate a higher level. Your best bet is to start out with the weaker products and work your way up. Those with very sensitive skin should stick with the weaker products.

POSSIBLE BENEFITS

Skin Rejuvenator. Alpha-hydroxy acids have been found to loosen the 'cement' binding cells on the skin, permitting the top layer of dead cells to shed more evenly and rapidly, thus revealing smoother, fresher-looking skin underneath. Many studies confirm that alpha-hydroxy acids are an effective treatment against extremely dry, flaky skin. They have also been used to treat conditions such as psoriasis. In addition, studies show that these skin products may help erase fine lines and age spots, and improve the tone and texture of the skin.

There is some controversy in the medical community over the effectiveness of over-the-counter alpha-hydroxy acid preparations. The more potent products used by dermatologists are more effective, but they are also more costly and can cause more skin irritation. Many people, however, find that the milder products are surprisingly effective at a fraction of the cost.

ASCORBIC ACID (VITAMIN C)

FACTS If you want to live longer, take your vitamin C. Recent studies suggest that vitamin C supplements (in addition to a diet rich in vitamin C foods) may prevent premature death from heart disease, and may even be a more important factor in preventing fatal heart attacks than maintaining a low cholesterol level or eating a low fat diet.

Vitamin C is also a potent antioxidant and works with other antioxidants in the body to help prevent damage from free radicals that may lead to various forms of cancer.

Vitamin C, a water soluble vitamin, is necessary for the formation of collagen, the substance that binds together the cells of connective tissue. Collagen is also essential for the production of new cells and tissues.

Vitamin C is reputed to be good for colds—in fact several studies show that although vitamin C cannot prevent the common cold, it can lessen its severity by decreasing the histamine level in your bloodstream by up to 40 per cent. Histamine causes the runny nose and watery eyes associated with colds and allergies.

19

Good natural sources of vitamin C include mango, kiwi fruit, grapefruit, broccoli, cantaloupe, strawberry, sweet red pepper, sweet potato, snow peas and orange juice.

THE RIGHT AMOUNT   The RDA for vitamin C is 60 mg, for smokers 100 mg, but about half of the UK population does not get even 60 mg of this vitamin daily. Studies suggest that the RDA is much too low and I recommend 1000 mg daily of calcium ascorbate (the gentlest form of vitamin C for your stomach.) Although many people can tolerate up to 10,000 mg of vitamin C daily, in some individuals an excess can cause dry nose, diarrhoea, excess urination and skin rashes.

POSSIBLE BENEFITS

Heart Disease. Researchers at the University of California looked at the vitamin C intakes and death rates of more than 11,000 men and women. The study showed a dramatic decline in death from heart disease among men with the highest vitamin C intake—especially among those who took a vitamin C supplement. Merely obtaining the RDA for vitamin C through food did not seem to offer any protection against heart disease. The results were similar among women, but less dramatic.

There are several reasons why vitamin C may protect against heart disease. Other studies have shown that this vitamin is particularly effective in intercepting oxidants before they can attack blood lipids. Many researchers believe that when LDL or 'bad' cholesterol is oxidised, it promotes the formation of plaque which can cause atherosclerotic lesions in arteries.

Raises Blood Glutathione. Glutathione is one of the most important antioxidants produced in the body. It protects cells from damage inflicted by hydroperoxides (free radicals) a natural byproduct of metabolism. Low levels of serum glutathione have been associated with cell damage, depressed immunity and premature ageing. A recent study conducted at Arizona State University showed how glutathione levels fluctuate in humans according to vitamin C intake. People on diets poor in vitamin C had low levels of glutathione, but when given a supplement

20

of 500 mg of vitamin C, their blood glutathione levels bounced back to normal.

Cancer Fighter. Many studies have investigated the association of dietary vitamin C and various forms of cancer. We know from these studies that dietary intake of vitamin C (through food, notably fruits and vegetables) appears to offer some protection against cancers of the lung, cervix, pancreas, mouth, throat, oesophagus, colon and stomach. In particular, vitamin C may protect against cancers of the stomach because it blocks the formation of nitrosamines in the stomach, which are potential carcinogens.

There is also some evidence that vitamin C may help to protect against breast cancer, especially in postmenopausal women.

Prevents Cataracts. Cataract, an opaque covering that can form on the lens of the eye, is particularly common among people over 50. Researchers at the Laboratory for Nutrition and Vision Research at the USDA Human Nutrition Center at Tufts University suggest that cataracts may be caused by cellular damage due to oxidation. For example, when vitamin C was added to the diet of guinea pigs, their eyes showed less oxidative damage after exposure to ultraviolet light than those of guinea pigs not given vitamin C. In human studies, adults taking antioxidant supplements (including vitamin C) were less likely to develop cataracts than those not taking vitamins.

PERSONAL ADVICE   Here's one supplement that everyone should be taking!

ASHWAGANDA

FACTS   The root of the ashwaganda plant is an important healing herb that is commonly used in the Ayurveda, the traditional herbal medicine of India. Ashwaganda is a small shrub belonging to the nightshade family which includes potatoes, tomatoes and aubergine.

Although many Western natural healers advise people with arthritis to avoid eating nightshade plants, in the Ayurveda ashwaganda has long been prescribed to treat this condition. Recent studies show that ashwaganda may indeed be effective against arthritis, and may also be a potent weapon against cancer. Over the last few years the Ayurveda has become very popular in the West because of its emphasis on the prevention of disease.

THE RIGHT AMOUNT   Ashwaganda teas and other herbal products are available at health food shops. Ashwaganda is included in many herbal formulae for arthritis. Drink one to two cups of the tea daily, or follow the directions on the package.

CAUTION   Ashwaganda contains some compounds which may be harmful at very high amounts. Do not exceed the recommended dose.

POSSIBLE BENEFITS

Arthritis. Several Indian studies have confirmed that ashwaganda has anti-inflammatory activity and can help reduce some of the stiffness and swelling associated with arthritis in both animals and humans. In one recent study performed at the University of Poona in Pune, 42 patients with osteoarthritis were given a herbal formula which included ashwaganda (among other herbs) and zinc complex. For three months the patients took the herbal formula; then, after a two-week period to allow the herbs to wear off, they were given a placebo for a further three months. The results: while on the herbal formula, the patients experienced a significant drop in severity of pain and stiffness.

Cancer Fighter. Several animal studies have shown that extract of ashwaganda root can inhibit the growth of tumours in laboratory mice.

ASPIRIN

FACTS   In 1958, when I started my pharmacy training, if anyone had suggested that aspirin—the 'wonder drug' of the nineteenth century—would be touted as a 'hot' anti-ageing drug at the dawn of the twenty-first, he or she would have been laughed out of the classroom. However, good old aspirin, chemically known as acetyl salicylic acid, holds great promise for the future as a protector against both cancer and heart disease.

Aspirin is actually a synthetic version of salicum, a natural derivative of the bark of the white willow tree, a long-established herbal remedy for headaches, fever and arthritis. Until recently, aspirin has been used as an analgesic to treat daily aches and pains. However, recent studies suggest that this drug may be underutilised.

THE RIGHT AMOUNT To help prevent certain forms of cancer and heart disease, I recommend taking one baby aspirin (about 81 mg) every day. Your doctor may suggest a higher dose if you are at risk of developing heart disease or certain forms of cancer.

CAUTION Do not take aspirin on a regular basis without first checking with your doctor. People with bleeding disorders or who are taking blood-thinning drugs should steer clear of aspirin unless advised otherwise by their doctors. Aspirin can be very irritating to the stomach and in some people can cause bleeding and ulcers. People on aspirin should be closely monitored by their doctors for gastrointestinal bleeding or other problems. If untreated, bleeding ulcers can cause severe problems, including death.

POSSIBLE BENEFITS

Heart Disease and Stroke. Will an aspirin a day keep the cardiologist away? There is strong evidence that it just might. Aspirin is a blood thinner—that is, it prevents the clumping together of blood platelets, tiny circulating discs that play a key role in the formation of blood clots. A majority of heart attacks and strokes are caused by blood clots forming in arteries that were already narrowed due to atherosclerotic lesions (deposits of lipids and other cells). By preventing the formation of blood clots, aspirin may play a significant role in preventing heart attacks and stroke. Consider the results of several recent studies:

- A study of 22,000 healthy male doctors given 325 mg of aspirin (the amount in one adult tablet) daily for five years had 44 per cent fewer heart attacks than those who did not take the aspirin.
- A study of 87,678 female nurses over eight years found a 30 per cent reduction in risk of first heart attack among women who took one to six aspirin per week. In this study, the aspirin was not prescribed, rather these women took aspirin on their own to treat headaches or musculoskeletal pain.
- In yet another study of more than 1,000 recovering heart patients performed at the Multicenter Study of Myocardial Ischemia in New Orleans, those who were not taking aspirin were three times more likely to have a fatal heart attack than those who were on the drug.

Cancer Fighter. Aspirin is an anti-inflammatory drug. It blocks the formation of prostaglandins, hormonelike substances in the body that can trigger an inflammatory response. By quelling inflammation, aspirin can help to relieve the pain of arthritis and bring down a fever. Prostaglandins are also believed to promote the growth of cancerous tumours, so by nipping them in the bud aspirin may indirectly be a potent cancer fighter.

Based on a study of more than 635,000 people performed by the American Cancer Society, those who took aspirin were at significantly lower risk of dying from digestive tract cancers (oesophagus, stomach, rectum and colon). In fact, men and women who took aspirin at least 16 times a month were 40 per cent less likely to die from these cancers than those who did not. The risk was lowest among men and women who used aspirin regularly for ten years or more.

ASTRAGALUS

FACTS   As we age our immune systems become weakened, leaving us more vulnerable to infection and disease. A handful of vitamins and herbs may help to keep the immune system functioning at optimum levels, and astragalus may be one of them. For centuries, oriental healers have used this herb to treat a wide variety of ailments, ranging from diabetes to high blood pressure, and have also prescribed it as an immune booster that strengthens the Wei Ch'i or defensive energy of the body. Western scientists are now beginning to acknowledge that this herb may indeed have a positive effect on immunity.

Astragalus, which is native to China and Japan, is being studied in the United States as a possible treatment for AIDS, a disease characterised by the breakdown of the immune system.

THE RIGHT AMOUNT   Astragalus is available in capsule form in health food shops. Take one to three (400 mg) capsules daily.

POSSIBLE BENEFITS

Immune Booster. Research by Dr G. Mavligit of the University of Texas Medical Center in Houston found that a purified extract of astragalus stimulates T-cells (one of the key white cells of the immune system) in healthy animals and helps to normalise the immune systems of cancer patients with impaired immunity due to chemotherapy. Other studies have shown that astragalus can stimulate the production of interferon, a protein, produced in cells, that fights against viral invasion. In fact, according to one Chinese study, patients given astragalus root developed fewer colds than patients not given the root, and when they did get a cold they had it for a significantly shorter amount of time than untreated patients.

Heart Disease. In China, astralagus has been used to treat cardiovascular disease. Animal studies show that this herb can lower blood pressure and may help to prevent heart attacks by improving the flow of blood to the heart.

BETA-CAROTENE

FACTS   Beta-carotene, one of 600 or so naturally occurring plant compounds in the carotene family, is also known as pro-vitamin A. Some of the beta-carotene we eat is converted to vitamin A as the body needs it. Although beta-carotene is an antioxidant, when it is converted to vitamin A it loses much of its antioxidant properties.

Of all the phytochemicals, beta-carotene is one of the most widely studied. Numerous studies show that people who eat diets rich in beta-carotene have lower levels of cancer and coronary artery disease than those who do not.

Good food sources of beta-carotene include apricots, sweet potato, broccoli, cantaloupe, pumpkin, carrot, mangoes, peaches and spinach.

THE RIGHT AMOUNT   The RDA for vitamin A is 2500 iu or 750 re (retinol equivalent). A 3 mg dose of beta-carotene is equal to 5000 iu of vitamin A. Although vitamin A can be toxic at doses higher than 25,000 iu daily, beta-carotene is not believed to be toxic even at high doses. In fact, many studies have used dosages as high as 50 mg of beta-carotene without any problem.

Most scientists agree that we need at least 6 mg of beta-carotene daily—many recommend as much as 14 mg daily. Most people ingest about 2 mg.

Beta-carotene supplements are sold individually. In addition, beta-carotene is included in most antioxidant formulae, as well as most multivitamins.

Beta-carotene comes in two forms which vary slightly in molecular structure: all-trans and the 9-cis beta-carotene. The 9-cis form may be better absorbed by the body.

POSSIBLE BENEFITS

Cancer Fighter. A study presented at the 1994 American Cancer Society Science Writers' Seminar showed that beta-carotene can reverse pre-cancerous sores in the mouth, suggesting that it could play a role in preventing oral cancers. People with oral lesions were given 60 mg of beta-carotene daily. After six months, most of the patients experienced a 50 per cent reduction or more in the number of mouth lesions, thus reducing their risk of developing oral cancers.

Medical journals worldwide are filled with studies linking low beta-carotene intake and/or low blood levels of beta-carotene to an increased risk of many different forms of cancer, including cancers of the breast, cervix, lung, stomach, colon and rectum, bladder, mouth and oesophagus. For example, in a recent study, researchers in Buffalo, New York, found that women with breast cancer had lower concentrations of plasma beta-carotene than those who were cancer free. A major study in Latin American countries performed by the American National Cancer Institute suggested that a high beta-carotene intake was associated with a 32 per cent reduction in cervical cancer.

Heart Disease. Recently, many researchers have begun to believe that atherosclerosis (the clogging of arteries with plaque) may be caused by the oxidation of LDL or 'bad' cholesterol. Several studies have shown that beta-carotene can significantly block the oxidation of LDL cholesterol, at least in test tubes. Population studies confirm that people with a high intake of beta-carotene have a lower rate of heart disease than those with a low intake. For example, ongoing research in the Nurses' Health Study shows that by eating even one serving of fruits or vegetables daily, you can reduce your risk of heart attack and stroke. Women in the study who took 15–20 mg of beta-carotene daily had a 22 per cent reduced risk of heart attack and a 40 per cent reduced risk of stroke.

Immune Protector. Ultraviolet A light from the sun not only promotes wrinkles and skin cancer, but may have harmful effects on the immune system. Researchers at Cornell University and Hoffman-LaRouche tested beta-carotene's ability to protect the immune system from UVA damage. In the study, 24 healthy men were put on a low-carotene diet for 28 days. Part of the group took a 30 mg supplement of beta-carotene; the others took a placebo. The whole group was exposed to UVA light several times over the next two weeks. Blood tests were then taken to measure the amount of beta-carotene and the ability of the blood to respond to various disease-causing antigens. The results: those on the beta-carotene showed a stronger immune response than those on the placebo.

Another study involved 21 patients who tested positive for the HIV virus but did not show any signs of AIDS. These patients were given either 180 mg of beta-carotene daily or a placebo. Of the 17 patients who actually completed the four-week study, the beta-carotene group showed significant increases in several blood factors that help to fight infection. This is not to suggest that beta-carotene is a cure for AIDS; however, it does appear to strengthen the body's immune system.

Cataracts. Several studies have shown that antioxidants in general, and beta-carotene in particular, can protect against the formation of cataracts. According to the Nurses' Health Study, women who eat a diet rich in beta-carotene have a 39 per cent lower risk of cataracts than those with a low beta-carotene intake.

PERSONAL ADVICE Eat a diet rich in dark green leafy vegetables and yellow and orange fruits and vegetables to get the broad spectrum benefits of beta-carotene.

BILBERRY

FACTS The eyes are one of the most important—and most vulnerable—organs, particularly as we age. Reading glasses have become one of the hallmarks of middle age. Later in life, cataracts (growths which cloud the lens of one or both eyes) and macular degeneration (which causes a blur or blind spot in the field of vision) are common occurrences which may be treated surgically, although not always successfully. At any age, exposure to TV and computer screens can lead to eye strain. Bilberry, a common herb, is one of the few known substances that may help preserve precious vision.

Bilberry grows wild in Europe and Asia and is similar to the North American blueberry. As with most other herbs, although US scientists have ignored bilberry, serious research on the fruit has been done in Europe, where it is widely used to treat and prevent a number of different disorders.

Bilberry contains biologically active compounds called anthocyanosides which may have many positive effects on the body.

THE RIGHT AMOUNT Bilberry is available in capsule form. Take one capsule up to three times daily.

POSSIBLE BENEFITS

Eyes. For centuries herbal healers have used bilberry to treat eye problems. During World War II, RAF pilots who munched on sandwiches made of bilberry jam before flying their night missions claimed that the jam improved their night vision. Later, studies confirmed that bilberry does indeed enhance eyesight. In 1964, French researchers found that bilberry improved the adaptation to dark after exposure to bright light. However, the improvement was short-lived: within 24 hours after taking the bilberry, the beneficial effects had worn off. Later, animal studies revealed that bilberry anthocyanosides work by accelerating the regeneration of retinol purple (visual purple), a substance that is required for good eyesight, especially at night.

Strengthens Capillaries. Anthocyanosides have been used as a treatment for capillary fragility (capillaries are extremely narrow blood vessels), a condition which may increase the risk of infection, traumatic injury and vascular disease. In addition, studies show that bilberry may be a useful tool in preventing vascular disease which can cause serious circulatory problems in diabetics.

BIOFLAVONOIDS

FACTS Bioflavonoids are a group of about 500 compounds that provide colour to citrus fruits and vegetables. Once regarded as little more than food dye, many of these compounds are now being investigated by the American National Cancer Institute for their potential disease-preventive properties.

Some bioflavonoids are potent antioxidants and are believed to work in conjunction with vitamin C—each may enhance the function of the other. They also work with vitamin C to keep connective tissues healthy. Bioflavonoids are sometimes referred to as vitamin P, short for capillary permeability factor, because they improve the strength of small blood vessels or capillaries. When the capillary walls are weakened, materials from the blood can penetrate the tissues, which may result in easy bruising or haemorrhaging.

One bioflavonoid, rutin, has been used successfully to treat bleeding gums. Bioflavonoids are used by natural healers to treat allergies and asthma. Synthetic versions of these compounds are used in prescription medications for asthma.

The best food sources of bioflavonoids include the white pith and segment part of citrus fruits, apricots, buckwheat, red and yellow onions, blackberries, cherries, rose hips, tea and apples.

THE RIGHT AMOUNT There is no RDA for bioflavonoids. These compounds are not considered a true vitamin because no deficiency state has been established. They are usually available in supplements with vitamin C (the normal combination is 500 mg vitamin C to 100 mg bioflavonoids.) Various bioflavonoids are also sold separately as supplements.

POSSIBLE BENEFITS

Heart Disease. Bioflavonoids appear to offer protection against heart disease. Researchers in Holland evaluated the diets of 805 men aged 65 to 84. The group who consumed the highest amounts of bioflavonoids in their diets had the lowest rate of heart disease. Researchers speculated that the antioxidant action of bioflavonoids may prevent the oxidising of LDL cholesterol, which can cause atherosclerosis.

Cancer Fighter. Recent studies show that some bioflavonoids may inhibit the action of carcinogens, thus blocking the initiation of cancerous changes in the cells. In addition, the antioxidant properties of bioflavonoids may also help to prevent cancers caused by oxidative damage. (For example, quercetin, which is found in red and yellow onions, has been shown to inhibit the activity of several carcinogens and tumour promoters.)

Anti-viral. Some bioflavonoids have been shown to have antiviral activity, especially in combination with vitamin C. For instance, in one study, a combination of 100 mg of vitamin C and 100 mg of bioflavonoids dramatically accelerated the healing of cold sores caused by the *Herpes labialis* virus. In test tube studies, quercetin and vitamin C were effective against the Coxsackie virus and the common cold.

PERSONAL ADVICE Bioflavonoids in combination with vitamin D may help to relieve hot flushes associated with menopause. Take 1000 mg of bioflavonoids and 400–800 ius of vitamin D daily.

BORON

FACTS Until recently, boron was not considered to be of particular importance. There is no RDA for boron—like other trace minerals, it is needed by the body in minuscule amounts. However, boron may prove the adage that good things come in small packages. Although the body only needs a tiny quantity of this mineral, it may play a big role in helping to prevent osteoporosis, and may even help your brain to work better.

Boron is found in most fruits and vegetables; however, dried fruits (prunes, apricots) are the best source.

THE RIGHT AMOUNT Take 3 mg daily (do not exceed 10 mg daily). I recommend boron supplements in the form of sodium borate. Boron works best if taken in a good vitamin and mineral supplement including calcium, magnesium, manganese and riboflavin.

POSSIBLE BENEFITS

Strong Bones. One in four women are likely to develop osteoporosis, characterised by the thinning or wearing away of bones, which makes them more vulnerable to breaks and fractures. Complications from osteoporosis are a leading cause of death among the elderly. Recent studies suggest that boron may play an important role in helping the body to retain bone mass. Under the direction of Dr Forrest H. Nielson, Supervisory Nutritionist, USDA Agricultural Research Services, researchers tested the effect of boron depletion on 12 postmenopausal women. For 119 days, women were given 2,000 calorie diets very low in boron (0.25 mg). The women were later given the same diet supplemented with 3 mg of boron for 48 days. Researchers found that the boron supplement reduced the loss of calcium and magnesium in the urine, both of which are minerals that are needed to help build strong bones. In addition, the boron supplement dramatically elevated levels of serum oestrogen and ionised calcium. This is important because women who develop osteoporosis tend to have low serum oestrogen levels and low levels of ionised calcium.

A subsequent study of boron depletion in men and women yielded similar results. In both sexes, boron appears to help the body maintain the essential minerals necessary to prevent bone loss.

Brain Function. In a USDA study of boron depletion in men and women aged 45-plus, subjects on a low boron diet displayed impaired mental functioning when asked to perform simple tasks such as counting and tapping. Electroencephalograms (a test which measures the electrical activity of the brain) showed that low dietary boron, in the researcher's own words, 'depressed mental alertness'.

BROMELAIN

FACTS Bromelain is an enzyme found in raw pineapple. For several decades health food enthusiasts have used it to treat many different ailments, ranging from indigestion to arthritis, and it is beginning to enjoy widespread acceptance among older 'baby-boomers' who prefer nature's pharmacy to the synthetic brews found in the conventional pharmacy.

THE RIGHT AMOUNT Fresh, raw pineapple is a good source of bromelain, although supplements offer a more concentrated form of this enzyme. Bromelain is included in many digestive aid formulae sold in health food shops, and bromelain tablets are also available. Take one to three daily.

POSSIBLE BENEFITS

Digestive Aid. Bromelain helps to break down protein. As we age, a decrease in hydrochloric acid production can prevent the proper digestion and absorption of protein and a daily bromelain supplement may help to compensate for the loss of HCL.

Anti-inflammatory. Bromelain has anti-inflammatory properties which may help to reduce the discomfort caused by rheumatoid arthritis. There have not been many clinical studies to confirm this, but there is a good deal of anecdotal evidence. Because of these anti-inflammatory properties, bromelain is also used by athletes to prevent the soreness that accompanies a strenuous work-out. It is also believed to facilitate the healing of sports injuries.

Antiallergic. Bromelain can also help to alleviate allergic symptoms by mediating the inflammatory response that triggers an allergic attack.

BURDOCK

FACTS   Called *lappa* in parts of Europe and *gobo* in Japan, the burdock root enjoys worldwide recognition as a mild, nourishing herb that may help to keep the body working well from childhood to old age.

For thousands of years burdock root and leaves have been used to treat rheumatism, gout and skin disorders such as psoriasis. The herb has also been used by traditional healers as a cancer treatment (along with other herbs) and is considered to be an excellent digestive aid and liver tonic.

The herbalist Christopher Hobbs includes burdock in his list of 'adaptogens', which he defines as important herbs that can be taken daily without any side effects and help 'restore to balance all bodily systems.' Herbalist Rosemary Gladstar, author of *Herbal Healing for Women*, prescribes burdock for women in all stages of life.

The Japanese, who have the longest life span of any nationality in the world, frequently eat burdock root. Fresh burdock root is available at some greengrocers, Asian supermarkets and specialist food shops.

THE RIGHT AMOUNT   Burdock root is available in capsules. Take one to three daily.

POSSIBLE BENEFITS

Cancer Fighter. Burdock root extracts have been shown to inhibit tumour growth in animal studies.

Liver. Burdock leaves and root are believed to stimulate the production of bile by the liver. Bile is essential for the breakdown of fats.

Fights Infection. Studies show that compounds in burdock have antibacterial and antifungal properties.

PERSONAL ADVICE According to folklore, a lotion made from the leaves of this plant should be massaged into the scalp to prevent hair from falling out.

BUTCHER'S BROOM

FACTS Butcher's broom is one of the most popular anti-ageing herbs in Europe. It contains compounds called ruscogins that are similar in structure to steroids. French studies have shown that butcher's broom is a vasoconstrictor: it strengthens veins and reduces capillary fragility (capillaries are tiny blood vessels.)

THE RIGHT AMOUNT Butcher's broom is available in capsule form. Take 400 mg daily. Suppositories and ointments are available to treat haemorrhoidal flare-ups. Use as directed.

POSSIBLE BENEFITS

Varicose Veins. Blood flows to the heart via a network of arteries, and away from the heart via a network of veins. Unlike arteries which are thick and strong, veins are weaker and less elastic, and are therefore prone to develop certain problems. When veins become swollen and enlarged, they are called varicosities. Varicose veins usually occur in the legs, where blood tends to pool due to poor circulation. Many women over 40 develop varicose veins in the legs.

Haemorrhoids—swollen anal veins—are a common ailment

of middle age. Overweight and chronic constipation are risk factors for developing haemorrhoids.

Many European studies show that when used over an extended period of time, butcher's broom can greatly relieve the pain and swelling associated with varicose veins and haemorrhoids. In Europe this herb is commonly used for these problems.

CALCIUM

FACTS For a lifetime of strong bones, normal blood pressure and even some protection against cancer, calcium is just what the doctor ordered. Unfortunately, most people do not take enough of this mineral, and the results can be devastating in later life.

Calcium is used for building strong teeth and bones and in maintaining bone strength. It is also important for maintenance of cell membranes, blood clotting and muscle absorption.

Good sources of calcium are low fat dairy products, kale, broccoli, tinned salmon or sardines with bones and calcium-fortified fruit juice.

THE RIGHT AMOUNT The RDA for adults up to 25 is 1200 mg, and from 25 to 50, 800 mg. Most women and younger men consume less than half the calcium they need. Postmenopausal women should get 1500 mg of calcium daily, but few do.

It may be difficult to obtain all the calcium you need through diet alone. I recommend using a non-natural source, such as calcium lactate, calcium gluconate and calcium carbonate. Vitamin D helps facilitate calcium absorption.

POSSIBLE BENEFITS

Strong Bones. Osteoporosis is a condition characterised by low bone mass and increased susceptibility to fractures, primarily in the hip, spine and wrist. Postmenopausal women are particularly vulnerable to this problem, in fact one third of all women in their 80s will experience a hip fracture. Recent studies suggest that calcium may play a leading role in helping to reduce bone loss that can lead to osteoporosis.

In a recent French study, more than 1,600 postmenopausal women were given 1200 mg of calcium and 800 iu of vitamin D daily for 18 months. Another group was given a placebo. The results: a 43 per cent reduction in hip fractures among the vitamin-supplemented group. Moreover, in the group on calcium and vitamin D, bone density rose 2.7 per cent on the hip, while density dropped 4.6 per cent in the untreated group.

Calcium alone may not be enough to prevent osteoporosis— other studies show that exercise may also play a preventive role, as well as postmenopausal hormone replacement therapy (HRT). In fact, for some women, a combination of all three may be their strongest defence against this bone-breaking disease.

Lowers Blood Pressure. High blood pressure—that is, pressure over 140/90—is associated with an increased risk of heart disease and stroke. (The top number, systolic pressure, is generated when the heart contracts and pushes blood through the artery. The bottom number, the diastolic pressure, is the pressure in the arteries when the heart muscle relaxes between beats.) Several studies have established that calcium supplements can lower blood pressure. A 13-year California study of 6,634 men and women showed that people who consumed 1000 mg of calcium daily reduced their risk of developing hypertension by 20 per cent. Another study of children (the Framingham Children's Study) revealed that the children who ate the most calcium-rich foods had the lowest blood pressure. As we age, blood pressure tends to rise; therefore adding calcium to your diet may help to prevent you developing serious hypertension.

Cancer Protection. Several studies have linked low intake of calcium and vitamin D with an increased risk of colon cancer. For example, a 19-year study of more than 1,500 men in Chicago found that an intake of more than 375 mg of calcium daily (roughly the amount in one glass of milk) was associated with a 50 per cent reduction in the rate of colon cancer, as compared to an intake of over 1200 mg which was associated with a 75 per cent decrease in colon cancer. Researchers suspect that calcium may bind with fatty acids, thus preventing them from irritating the colon walls. Low intakes of calcium may also increase the rate of excretion of vitamin D, which also appears to play a role in helping to prevent colon cancer. Think of it this way: two cups of skimmed milk or calcium-fortified orange juice, and two servings of low fat yogurt may be all that it takes to prevent this potentially lethal cancer.

CAPSAICIN

FACTS Capsaicin (also known as cayenne), a compound derived from hot chilli peppers, gives new meaning to the phrase 'hot hundred'. Capsaicin is the substance that gives chillies their unique bite. Hot chillies have been used in cooking for thousands of years, and herbal healers have prescribed them for various ailments ranging from asthma and arthritis to indigestion (contrary to popular belief, hot foods do not cause stomach distress in a healthy stomach, although they may irritate ulcers. In fact, chillies actually stimulate the production of saliva and gastric acids which aid digestion).

In recent years, capsaicin has gained the respect of traditional medical practitioners and, ironically, is now considered one of the most important 'new' compounds in medicine. Capsaicin has many different effects on the body, and some of them may indeed help to extend life. However, even if capsaicin does not promote longevity, I believe that it can, at the very least, improve the quality of life for older adults, especially for those in chronic pain.

THE RIGHT AMOUNT Capsaicin (cayenne) is available in many different forms including capsules, tea and ointment. Take one to three capsules daily, or drink one cup of tea daily. Capsaicin ointment may be used on the skin for relief of shingles and arthritic pain. Some people may find the ointment irritating, so check with your doctor before using it.

POSSIBLE BENEFITS

Heart Disease. In animal studies, capsaicin has had a favourable effect on blood lipid levels, which can help reduce the risk of heart disease and stroke. According to a 1987 study published in the *Journal of Bioscience*, rats fed a diet high in capsaicin experienced a significant reduction in blood triglycerides and LDL or 'bad' cholesterol. (Triglycerides over 190 mg/dl for women and over 400 mg/dl for men are believed to increase the risk of heart attack.)

Pain Relief. When you rub capsaicin cream on your skin, you immediately feel a hot, burning sensation that eventually tapers off. Recently, scientists have learned that capsaicin stimulates certain nerve cells to release a chemical called substance P which sends pain signals throughout the nervous system. Capsaicin quickly depletes the cells of substance P, thus temporarily blocking their ability to transmit any more pain impulses. Capsaicin skin cream is now used topically to treat various ailments, including shingles, a particularly painful rash caused by the reactivation of the chicken pox virus that often strikes older adults. Shingles usually disappears within three or four weeks, but in older adults or in people with weakened immune systems it can linger on in the form of post-herpetic neuralgia, a very painful and distressing ailment. A potent form of capsaicin cream is one of the few treatments that has offered any relief to the victims of post-herpetic neuralgia, and it has also been used quite effectively to treat diabetic neuropathy, a condition characterised by severe foot and ankle pain. Several over-the-counter creams containing capsaicin are also used to treat the pain and stiffness of arthritis. (If you use a cream containing capsaicin, be careful to avoid getting it in your eyes.)

Mood Enhancer. When you bite into a hot chilli pepper, you feel a rush of heat that can quite literally bring tears to your eyes. The body responds to this 'pain' by releasing endorphins, chemicals in the brain that have a pain-relieving effect similar to morphine. Capsaicin may be nature's way of helping you to beat the blues.

PERSONAL ADVICE   Cayenne tea can have a mild, stimulating effect. When you're feeling down, have a cup for a quick pick-me-up.

CENTELLA (GOTU-KOLA)

FACTS Although most people can maintain good health throughout their lifetime, there are times when an accident or illness may result in prolonged bed rest or reduced activity. Centella (also called Gotu Kola) can help you get back on your feet faster by preventing dangerous complications that can result during an extended period of inactivity.

THE RIGHT AMOUNT Centella is available in capsules or extract. Take one capsule up to three times daily. Mix five to ten drops of extract in a cup of liquid. Take up to three times daily.

CAUTION Do not use this herb during pregnancy. People with an overactive thyroid should avoid this herb.

POSSIBLE BENEFITS

Circulatory Disorders. Patients confined to bed may develop venous insufficiency, a condition that seriously impairs the flow of blood throughout the body, especially in the feet and legs. In some cases, the veins may become inflamed, resulting in phlebitis, a painful and potentially serious condition. Compounds in centella have been shown to strengthen and tone veins and capillaries, and may help prevent circulatory problems. In addition, studies show that centella has been used successfully to treat patients suffering from problems related to venous insufficiency.

Wound Healing. Used externally or taken internally, centella can accelerate the healing of wounds, skin ulcers and other sores.

PERSONAL ADVICE According to herbalist Christopher Hobbs, legend has it that if you eat a leaf of centella each day, your life span will be extended one thousand years.

CHOLINE

FACTS Thousands of years ago, Chinese healers recommended foods such as eggs and meat for mental alertness, and foods such as fruits and grains for a more relaxed state. Until recently, modern psychiatry dismissed such notions as moonshine, but we now know that the chemicals in foods can indeed have a profound effect on our thought processes and mental well-being.

For example, egg yolks contain a compound called phosphatidylcholine, which is a major source of choline in the body. Recent studies suggest that choline may prove to be a 'memory tonic'.

The brain consists of millions of tiny neurons or cells which are connected by long tendrils called axons. The cells 'talk' to each other via chemicals called neurotransmitters. The brain uses choline to make acetylcholine, a neurotransmitter that plays a role in memory function.

Other good food sources of choline include soya beams, cabbage, peanuts and cauliflower.

THE RIGHT AMOUNT Choline is available in tablet and liquid form at health food shops. Take 1000 mg daily.

POSSIBLE BENEFITS

Memory Booster. Some researchers believe that, as we age, we begin to produce less acetylcholine, or the acetylcholine that is produced is less efficient, which is why many older people become forgetful. There is some evidence that choline deficiency may result in memory loss. Alzheimer's patients have lower levels of choline than normal; however, attempts to reverse the condition with choline supplements have so far been ineffective. Some researchers believe, however, that choline supplementation may slow down memory loss.

In another study, a drug that interferes with acetylcholine was given to college students. The students began to show signs of forgetfulness similar to those seen among the elderly. In fact many common drugs, including antihistamines, antidepressants and antispasmodics, may block acetylcholine and can cause short-term memory loss. Older people in particular are especially vulnerable to drug-induced memory loss, and are quick to assume that lapses in memory are a natural part of the ageing process. Very often, memory is restored when the drugs are stopped.

CHROMIUM PICOLINATE

FACTS   When you were a child, nobody ever told you to 'Take your chromium or no dessert!' Now that you are *not* a child any more, I'd like to remind you to 'Take your chromium'. As we age, we need this mineral more than ever.

Chromium is a trace mineral that works with insulin to help the body utilise sugar and metabolise fat. Recent studies suggest that chromium protects against heart disease, diabetes and may even help to firm up flabby muscles. What's even more exciting is the fact that a preliminary study hints that chromium may improve longevity.

Chromium is found in broccoli, whole-wheat English muffins, brewer's yeast, meat, cheese and shellfish.

THE RIGHT AMOUNT   The RDA for chromium is up to 200 mcg daily. Dr Richard Anderson of the USDA's Human Nutrition Research Center—a leading authority on chromium—says that we need at least 50 mcg daily; however, he concedes that most people fall short of this amount. Studies show that serum chromium levels decrease with age, which means that adults over 50 are often short on chromium.

Pure chromium supplements are not well absorbed by the body, but when chromium is combined with picolinic acid, it is better utilised by the body. I recommend taking a minimum of 200 mcg of chromium picolinate daily.

POSSIBLE BENEFITS

Improves Glucose Tolerance. Insulin helps the body to metabolise or break down glucose, or blood sugar, in a form that can be utilised by cells for energy. Animal studies show that

41

chromium helps regulate the release of insulin by acting on insulin-producing cells or beta cells. Beta cells in the pancreas manufacture and store insulin until a rising blood sugar level signals to them to release it. In a USDA study, one group of laboratory rats was fed a chromium-rich diet; the other was fed a chromium-deficient diet. Each group of rats was given a glucose solution to stimulate insulin. The rats fed the chromium-deficient diet secreted up to 50 per cent less insulin during the test than the rats given the chromium-sufficient diet. Based on this study, it appears as if chromium directly stimulates the production of insulin as the body needs it.

Human studies show that chromium supplements can normalise blood sugar levels in half the people with high blood sugar.

As people age, there is a tendency to develop type II diabetes mellitus, a condition characterised by high blood glucose levels, often caused by the body's failure to produce enough insulin. Researchers are hopeful that chromium may help to perk up insulin production in older adults, thus reducing the risk of developing this form of diabetes.

Lowers Blood Lipids. Several studies have shown that chromium can cut serum cholesterol levels and triglycerides, another form of blood lipid that may help to promote heart disease. In a study published in *The Western Journal of Medicine*, 28 volunteers with elevated cholesterol (220 to 320 mg/dl) were given either 200 mcg of chromium picolinate supplement or a placebo. After a six-week period, those on the chromium showed an average seven per cent drop in cholesterol, thus reducing their risk of heart disease by 14 per cent. LDL or 'bad' cholesterol levels dipped by more than ten per cent.

Muscle Builder. Chromium picolinate supplements are being promoted as a new and safe way to build muscle. Several studies have shown that supplements of chromium picolinate can increase muscle mass; however, it only works for people who exercise regularly. So if you want to firm up the flab, take a chromium supplement along with a sensible exercise regime. Sorry, couch potatoes, simply taking a chromium pill without exercise is not effective.

Longevity Drug. I've saved the best for last. A researcher at Bemidji State University in Minnesota fed chromium picolinate and two other chromium supplements to a small group of laboratory rats. The results: the rats on the chromium picolinate lived an average of one year longer than the rats on the other form of chromium. The chromium picolinate increased the average life span of the rats by one-third. Although we don't know whether chromium will help humans live longer, we do know that chromium can help prevent heart disease and diabetes, which can cut life short.

CINNAMON

FACTS Cinnamon has been a highly prized spice since ancient times and is used in many different cuisines. However, modern scientists are finding some new uses for this venerable spice. Recently, researchers have discovered that cinnamon (and a handful of other spices) may help control blood sugar levels by increasing the efficiency of insulin.

THE RIGHT AMOUNT Use this spice freely on cereal, fruit, yogurt, and even toast. I make a point of eating about a teaspoonful (5 ml) of cinnamon daily.

POSSIBLE BENEFITS

Diabetes. About one in four people have a genetic tendency to develop diabetes, a condition characterised by the inability of the body to metabolise and use foods properly. As a result, diabetics develop excessive amounts of blood sugar which is not utilised and is secreted into urine. In many cases the diabetic does not produce enough insulin, the hormone that helps to regular blood sugar. Insulin is produced by beta cells in the pancreas, and over time these cells can wear out. If untreated, diabetes may lead to severe complications, including heart disease. Most cases of diabetes occur later in life—in fact, a 65-year-old is 60 times more likely to develop diabetes than someone under 20. Even if you have a tendency to develop

43

diabetes, it is not inevitable that you will do so. Some doctors believe that the condition can be delayed or even avoided through proper diet. People who are overweight, especially women, are at much higher risk of developing diabetes than those of normal weight. A high fat, high calorie diet may overwhelm the beta cells, hastening the onset of diabetes. However, some foods and spices appear to help keep blood sugar levels under control. In recent test tube studies, cinnamon appeared significantly to increase the ability of insulin to metabolise glucose.

CITRUS

FACTS Will eating citrus fruits make you live longer? The American National Cancer Institute (NCI) is banking on it. The NCI is spending millions of dollars to study compounds found in orange, grapefruit, lemon and lime for their potential cancer-fighting properties.

Citrus fruits contain a virtual drug store of phytochemicals that may help to ward off disease. However, they are best known for being an excellent source of vitamin C, a potent antioxidant and enemy of the common cold. In addition, citrus fruits offer other important minerals including potassium (which controls blood pressure) and a fair amount of fibre, which is good for almost everything.

THE RIGHT AMOUNT Make one of your 'six a day' a citrus fruit.

POSSIBLE BENEFITS

Cancer Fighter. The NCI is investigating limonene, a citrus oil which has been shown to shrink mammary tumours in rats, and even better, prevented the growth of new tumours. Given the fact that breast cancer is so common, limonene may prove to be of great importance.

Citrus also contains compounds called bioflavonoids (also known as Vitamin P) which provide the yellow and orange colour of these fruits, and maybe much, much more. Some bioflavonoids are antioxidants that help prevent damage to cells inflicted by free radicals. Others help to prevent the spread of malignant cells throughout the body. Researchers hope that one day a form of bioflavonoid may be used to treat various forms of cancer.

In addition, citrus contains terpenes, compounds which help produce enzymes that deactivate carcinogens (and also limit the production of cholesterol) which may also prove to be a useful tool in the fight against cancer.

Heart Disease. Most heart attacks and strokes are caused by tiny blood clots that form in arteries that are already narrowed by atherosclerotic lesions. Citrus contains coumarins, natural blood thinners which may help prevent the formation of dangerous clots.

Pectin, a compound found in the pulpy membranes that separate individual sections in grapefruits and oranges, can lower blood cholesterol levels, thus reducing the risk of heart attack and stroke. Grapefruit pectin is the most effective. In a recent study at the University of Florida College of Medicine, people with high cholesterol levels were given grapefruit pectin (in a powdered form) daily. Within 16 weeks, the group's cholesterol dropped on average 7.6 per cent; LDL or 'bad' cholesterol was cut by ten per cent. Although the powdered form of grapefruit may be more potent than the natural pectin, researchers believe that whole grapefruit can also lower cholesterol, although perhaps not as much. However, since most people only eat the grapefruit sections and not the membrane containing the pectin, they miss out on the cholesterol-lowering benefit.

CLUB MOSS TEA

FACTS For centuries, Chinese healers have routinely prescribed a tea brewed from an oriental club moss (*Huperzia serrata*) to reverse memory loss in older people. Western scientists—who tended to dismiss all folk medicine—tried to no avail to concoct their own drug to reinvigorate people's memories.

In 1986, scepticism gave way to hope when researchers at the Shanghai Institute of Materia Medica reported that they had isolated natural compounds in club moss called huperzine A and huperzine B which, according to animal tests, helped to improve learning, memory retrieval and memory retention. (Huperzine A appeared to be the more effective.)

What Western scientists found most intriguing about huperzine was that it raised acetylcholine levels by inhibiting acetylcholinesterase, an enzyme which breaks down acetylcholine. Acetylcholine is a chemical found in the brain that is directly involved in memory and awareness. People with Alzheimer's disease, a life-threatening disorder characterised by severe memory loss and dementia, have lower than normal levels of acetylcholine. Since there is no treatment or cure for Alzheimer's, any compound that can raise acetylcholine levels is considered a potential weapon against this debilitating disease. Researchers at the Mayo Clinic in Jacksonville, Florida, have been studying huperzine as a potential drug for Alzheimer's. They have recently licensed the use of huperzine A to a pharmaceutical company which is seeking government permission to test the drug on humans.

THE RIGHT AMOUNT   Drink one or two cups of brewed club moss tea daily. There are several different types of club moss, so be sure that the tea is *Huperzia serrata*, and not some other species of club moss. Depending on where you live, getting the club moss may be a bit of a challenge; however, it should be available from major herbalists, and if you live in an area with a large Chinese population, check out some of the local specialist shops.

POSSIBLE BENEFITS

Memory Enhancer. Several animal studies confirm huperzine A's positive effect on memory. In one study, laboratory mice were taught how to run through an electric grid without getting a shock. After the training, the mice were given either an electric shock or a drug to induce amnesia. One group of mice was given huperzine immediately after the amnesia treatment, the other group was not. Twenty-four hours later, the mice were placed back on the electric grid to see how much they retained from their earlier training. The mice given huperzine performed significantly better than the untreated mice.

Will huperzine work as well on humans? There are some promising signs that it will. For example, Chinese studies have shown that huperzine can help to improve memory function in stroke victims. More studies are needed before we know for sure whether huperzine will offer relief from Alzheimer's disease, and whether it really is a potent memory tonic. However, in the meantime it can't hurt to include a cup or two of club moss tea in your daily diet.

COBALAMIN (VITAMIN B_{12})

FACTS Cobalamin, also known as Vitamin B_{12}, plays many important roles in the body. It aids in the production of red blood cells, is essential for the normal functioning of the nervous system, and also helps to metabolise protein and fat. Most recently, B_{12} has been touted as the 'brain vitamin', because a lack of this important vitamin can severely hamper mental agility in people of all ages. B_{12} deficiency is quite common among the elderly population—in fact as many as ten per cent of people over 60 may have low blood levels of this vitamin—and the results can be devastating.

B_{12} is found in meat, fish, eggs and dairy products.

THE RIGHT AMOUNT The RDA for B_{12} is 3 mcg for men and women. B_{12} is available in capsules, tablets, a nasal gel and a sublingual form that dissolves under the tongue.

POSSIBLE BENEFITS

Brain Booster. According to a recent study performed at the University Hospital of Maastricht in the Netherlands, otherwise healthy people with low blood levels of B_{12} did not perform as well in mental tests as people with higher blood levels of this vitamin, regardless of age.

Neurologic Symptoms in Older Adults. Vitamin B_{12} deficiency can cause severe neurologic and psychological symptoms in older people, ranging from numbness or tingling in the arms or legs (peripheral neuropathy) to balance problems, confusion and even dementia. If caught in time, many but not all of these problems can be reversed with B_{12} supplements. Unfortunately, many people are likely to dismiss confusion or erratic behaviour in the elderly as part of the natural ageing process and may not look for other causes. However, several studies show that B_{12} deficiency is extremely widespread among people over 60. In fact, according to a recent study of 100 people between the ages of 65 and 93, performed at New York Medical College, more than 21 had low B_{12} levels (of which two had peripheral neuropathy) and 16 had very low levels (of which three had peripheral neuropathy and one suffered from mental deterioration.)

Why is B_{12} deficiency so common among older adults? As people age, they are prone to develop a condition called atrophic gastritis, characterised by less gastric acid and increased amounts of bacteria in the upper small intestine and stomach. The combination of low levels of gastric acid and the presence of bacteria is believed to hamper the ability of the body to utilise the B_{12} in food. Antibiotics may be prescribed to reduce the level of bacteria, which may help increase the level of B_{12} derived from food. However, B_{12} supplements may be better absorbed than B_{12} bound to food.

If an older person shows signs of neurologic or psychological disturbances and other physical causes have been ruled out, he or she should be checked for B_{12} deficiency. In fact, some researchers now believe that every adult over 65 should be checked for B_{12} deficiency since the long-term consequences can be devastating.

PERSONAL ADVICE   I personally recommend the nasal gel or sublingual form, both of which bypass the stomach and are absorbed directly into the bloodstream.

COENZYME Q-10

FACTS An enzyme is a protein, found in living cells, which brings about chemical changes, and a coenzyme works with an enzyme to produce a particular reaction. Coenzyme Q-10 is found in every cell in the body and is essential in facilitating the process that provides cells with energy. As we age, levels of Coenzyme Q-10 begin to fall although exercise can help to raise them.

Coenzyme Q-10 can be synthesised by the body or obtained from food. Deficiency states may occur, particularly among the elderly.

Since 1974, Coenzyme Q-10 has been used successfully in Japan to treat heart disease—six million Japanese take it annually. Recent studies suggest that it may play a vital role in thwarting the ageing process and it can also increase your energy level, especially in people who do not exercise.

THE RIGHT AMOUNT Coenzyme Q-10 is available in capsules. Take 30 mg daily.

POSSIBLE BENEFITS

Heart Disease. Several studies have shown that Coenzyme Q-10 can increase stamina and reduce angina in heart patients. In one Japanese study, researchers selected ten men and two women with chronic unstable angina (chest pain) between the ages of 45 and 66. The twelve-week study was divided into three phases. In phase one patients were given a placebo. In phase two half the patients were given a placebo and the others were given 150 mg of Coenzyme Q-10 daily (50 mg three times a day.) In phase three the group on the placebo were given Coenzyme Q-10, and the group that had been given Coenzyme Q-10 were now given a placebo. During each phase, exercise tests were performed by patients on a treadmill. Patients on the Coenzyme Q-10 had fewer attacks of angina and were able to exercise longer than those not on the medication. In addition, those on the Coenzyme Q-10 required fewer nitroglycerine tablets (to relieve the pain of angina) than those on the placebo.

In Japan, Coenzyme Q-10 is used to treat congestive heart failure. It works by increasing the strength of the heart muscle. Studies have shown that it may lower blood pressure.

Antioxidant. Animal studies have shown that Coenzyme Q-10 inhibits lipid peroxidation, a process which may contribute to heart disease, premature ageing and even cancer. Antioxidants prevent cells from being damaged by free radicals, unstable oxygen molecules that can cause malignant changes in cells.

PERSONAL ADVICE   Coenzyme Q-10 is very effective in preventing toxicity from a large number of drugs used to treat cancer, high blood pressure and other diseases.

CRANBERRY

FACTS   Urinary tract infections (UTI), characterised by painful urination, blood or pus in the urine, fever, low back pain or cramps, are more common among older men and women. In men, enlargement of the prostate gland, a common condition affecting nearly half of all men over 50, can promote urinary infections. Postmenopausal women in particular suffer more UTI than younger women, due to vaginal dryness caused by lower oestrogen levels.

Once an infection has taken hold it must be properly treated with medication, and sometimes several drugs must be used before the infection clears up. However, studies have shown that cranberry juice can help prevent these annoying and painful infections from occurring in the first place.

THE RIGHT AMOUNT   Drink one to two glasses of cranberry juice daily. Cranberry concentrate is available in capsule form from health food shops. Take two to six capsules daily.

POSSIBLE BENEFITS

Prevents UTI. Urinary tract infections are caused by the *E. coli* bacterium which tends to adhere to the walls of the urinary tract. Recently, researchers at Alliance City Hospital in Ohio discovered that cranberry juice prevented E. *coli* from sticking to the endothelial cells of the urinary tract, so that the potentially dangerous bacterium was flushed out in the urine.

CRUCIFEROUS VEGETABLES

FACTS Population studies of dietary habits—so-called epidemiological studies—have shown that people who eat a diet high in cruciferous vegetables (cabbage, broccoli, brussels sprouts, kale, cauliflower) have lower rates of cancer than people who do not. Because of its possible role in fighting cancer, researchers at the American National Cancer Institute have begun investigating the cruciferous family to isolate its potential cancer-fighting properties.

THE RIGHT AMOUNT I recommend at least two servings of these vegetables daily.

POSSIBLE BENEFITS

Cancer Fighter. Researchers at the Institute for Hormone Research in New York have found that indoles, a group of phytochemicals in cruciferous vegetables, may be a powerful weapon against cancer. Indoles appear to alter the biological pathway that converts certain oestrogens into more potent forms that can trigger the growth of tumours in oestrogen-sensitive sites, such as the breast. Women with breast cancer tend to have higher blood oestrogen levels than normal, and any substance that controls the amount of oestrogen circulating in the bloodstream may have a protective effect against certain forms of breast cancer.

Researchers at Johns Hopkins School of Medicine in Baltimore recently found what may be an even more vigorous cancer fighter in cruciferous vegetables—sulphoraphane, a phytochemical that stimulates the action of protective enzymes which help the body fight against tumour growth (see Sulphoraphane, page 126). Indeed, one researcher has said that it may be one of the most potent protective agents against cancer discovered to date!

51

Antioxidant Boost. Cruciferous vegetables are rich in beta-carotene, vitamin C, selenium and vitamin E. These antioxidants may help to prevent the cellular damage caused by free radicals which may be responsible for many different forms of cancer and heart disease.

Fibre Boost. Cruciferous vegetables are excellent sources of fibre, which helps to prevent constipation and digestive diseases such as diverticulosis, but also may help to prevent cancer of the colon, breast, lung and cervix.

DANDELION

FACTS   To most suburbanites dandelions are just troublesome weeds, but to practitioners of herbal medicine they are a veritable gold mine. Herbalists have long used dandelions to treat liver ailments and digestive disorders and, like so many other herbs, they are now being rediscovered by men and women who are determined to maintain a lifetime of good health.

Dandelion is a very good source of beta-carotene and lutein, two members of the carotenoid family that may protect against certain forms of cancer.

THE RIGHT AMOUNT   Dandelion leaves can be eaten fresh in salads. Dandelion tea and capsules are available in health food shops. Drink one cup of tea daily or take one to three capsules daily. Dandelion is included in many herbal formulae designed to promote good digestion and improve liver function.

POSSIBLE BENEFITS

Liver. The liver weighs less than two kilos but it is worth its weight in gold several times over. It performs many vital jobs in the body, including the detoxification of poisons and impurities that may enter the bloodstream, the production of sex hormones, proteins and enzymes and the breakdown of fat. Animal studies show that dandelion extract can stimulate the production by the liver of bile which is essential for the metabolism of fat. Herbalists believe that dandelion is an overall tonic for the liver, generally improving its ability to function.

Digestive Aid. Dandelion, like other 'bitters', can help treat digestive problems such as wind and bloating. This herb can also help to prevent constipation.

Menopause Aid. Dandelion, which is rich in plant oestrogens, is often prescribed to relieve some of the discomfort of menopause caused by a sharp dip in oestrogen levels. It has a mild diuretic effect which can help eliminate menopausal water retention. However, unlike other diuretics, it is high in potassium and does not sap the body of this vital mineral.

DONG QUAI

FACTS Known in the West as dong quai and in the Far East as *tang keui*, this member of the angelica family is a highly esteemed anti-ageing herb. According to Ron Teeguarden, author of *Chinese Tonic Herbs*, it is the 'ultimate woman's tonic herb'. It is widely used throughout Asia to help ease the symptoms of menopause.

In younger women, dong quai is used to regulate menstrual disorders.

THE RIGHT AMOUNT Dong quai is available in tablet or capsule form and is included in many 'change of life' supplements sold in health food shops. Take two tablets or capsules twice daily.

POSSIBLE BENEFITS

Menopause. Chinese healers consider dong quai to be a hormone regulator that maintains hormones within normal levels. It contains hormonelike compounds that may relieve hot flushes, vaginal dryness and other symptoms of menopause and it is also rich in vitamin E, which may also explain why women may find it useful at this period of their lives. Dong quai has a mild, sedative effect which can help relieve stress.

Heart Disease. Studies show that this herb can lower blood pressure in both men and women and slow down the pulse rate.

Anaemia. Chinese women use dong quai as a 'blood builder'. It is a rich source of iron and may help to prevent iron deficiency anaemia.

Diabetes. Dong Quai has been shown to regulate blood sugar, thus helping to prevent high concentrations of glucose or blood sugar that can lead to diabetes.

PERSONAL ADVICE   Next time you are eating at a Cantonese Chinese restaurant, try ordering the dong quai duck.

ECHINACEA

FACTS   Echinacea is living proof that the more things change, the more they stay the same. Native Americans first used this beautiful purple cornflower as a remedy for toothaches, sore throats and even snake bites. European settlers brought echinacea back to Europe where it quickly became a popular herbal remedy. Around 1900, scientists who had studied the effect of echinacea on blood cultures recognised that this herb could boost the immune system by stimulating the production of white blood cells. Doctors as well as herbalists used echinacea to treat infection and cancer, but once antibiotics were discovered, interest waned in herbs such as this one. However, as interest in preventive medicine increased in the 1980s, researchers began to look for ways to keep people healthy. Anything that could bolster the immune system attracted attention, and interest in echinacea was revived. Today, as we approach the twenty-first century, echinacea is now being touted as a hot 'new' immuno-stimulant.

THE RIGHT AMOUNT   Echinacea is available in capsule, extract and as tablets at most health food shops and herb shops. Some preparations are made from the roots of the *Echinacea angustifolia* plant, others from the roots or leaves of *Echinacea purpurea*. Either form may be included in herbal preparations designed to boost the immune system.

I find that the capsules are the easiest. Take one capsule three times daily. If you prefer to use extract, mix 15 to 30 drops in liquid every three hours up to three times daily. Many of the active compounds in echinacea can be destroyed during processing. Freeze drying is the most effective way to preserve this herb's healing properties.

POSSIBLE BENEFITS

Anti-viral. Several studies have shown that echinacea prevents the formation of an enzyme called hyaluronidase, which destroys a natural barrier between healthy tissue and unwanted pathogenic organisms. Thus the herb helps cells maintain their natural line of defence against bacteria and viruses.

Several studies have shown that echinacea may be an effective treatment against colds, ear infections and flu. A recent German study of 180 patients between the ages of 18 and 60 showed that echinacea extract (four droppers daily) was significant in relieving the symptoms and duration of flu-like infections. (There is no reason to believe that capsules would not work as well.) Other European studies have shown that echinacea is useful in the treatment of ear infections in children.

In 1978, a study of echinacea in *Planta Medica* showed that a root extract destroyed both herpes and influenza virus.

Cancer Fighter. Several animal studies show that echinacea can inhibit the growth of certain types of tumours, probably by stimulating the production of key lymphocytes which, in turn, accelerate the body's own defences. Echinacea has also been used to restore normal immune function in patients receiving chemotheraphy.

Anti-fungal. At least one study has shown that echinacea (taken orally, and applied vaginally in cream form) may be an effective treatment against yeast infection (*Candida albicans*) a particularly persistent infection. Even better, this treatment appears to help prevent the infection from recurring.

ELLAGIC ACID

FACTS Ellagic acid, a polyphenolic compound found in fruit, is attracting a great deal of attention among cancer researchers because it appears to be a potent cancer fighter.

Strawberries, grapes and cherries are a good source of ellagic acid.

THE RIGHT AMOUNT There is no RDA for ellagic acid, and as yet not enough information is available to make it possible to recommend a specific amount. However, I advise people to eat at least one serving daily of a fruit containing this substance.

At the time of writing, ellagic acid is not available in supplement form. Even if it were, I generally advise people to try to get their phytochemicals through food whenever possible.

POSSIBLE BENEFITS

Cancer Fighter. Animal studies show that ellagic acid counteracts both synthetic and naturally occurring carcinogens, thus preventing healthy cells from turning cancerous. Ellagic acid is also an antioxidant which may block the destructive effects of free radicals.

Ellagic acid's ability to counteract carcinogens is very promising. For example, in one Japanese study, laboratory rats were fed a diet high in various polyphenolic compounds. One group was given ellagic acid exclusively. The rats were later exposed to a potent carcinogen to induce tongue cancer. All the rats on the various polyphenolic compounds had a reduced incidence of cancer, but those on the ellagic acid remained entirely cancer free. The researchers speculated that ellagic acid (and other polyphenols) may help to prevent cancer in other tissues, including skin, lung, liver and the oesophagus.

In another study, researchers tested the effect of ellagic acid on a nicotine-derived carcinogen found in cigarette smoke. The study revealed that the ellagic acid (and other polyphenols) blocked the carcinogenic effect of the nicotine compound on animal cells.

More research needs to be done to determine whether ellagic

acid will work in a similar way on humans. However, until the results are in, eating foods rich in ellagic acid cannot hurt, and it just might help.

FENUGREEK

FACTS Fenugreek is a herb used as a spice to flavour curry and chutney. Since ancient times it has been valued for its medicinal properties. Reputed to be an aphrodisiac, it has been used to treat impotency in men and discomfort associated with menopause in women. Modern scientists believe that fenugreek may play a role in helping to prevent or postpone adult onset diabetes.

THE RIGHT AMOUNT Fenugreek is available from health food shops as tea or in capsules. It is also included in many herbal formulae for women. Drink one or two cups of tea daily. One capsule may be taken three times daily.

CAUTION Do not use fenugreek during pregnancy.

POSSIBLE BENEFITS

Menopause. Fenugreek contains steroidal saponins similar to the sex hormones produced by the body, and therefore may play a role in regulating hormone levels. Herbal healers recommend fenugreek for hot flushes and depression associated with menopause.

Diabetes. According to USDA researcher Dr James A. Duke, fenugreek (along with a handful of other herbs and spices,) may help slow the onset of adult diabetes. Fenugreek seeds contain at least six different compounds that can help control blood sugar levels, thus preventing a sugar surge that may create problems for many older people who may not produce enough insulin, or may be insulin resistant.

FIBRE

FACTS There is one thing that advocates for alternative medicine and mainstream bodies like the British Medical Association can agree on: we should eat more fibre.

'Fibre' is a catch-all word for the non-nutritive food substances found in plants, which are not digested or absorbed by the body—so-called 'roughage'. Although there is compelling evidence that a diet high in fibre may help to ward off a number of deadly diseases, the Western diet is woefully low in fibre. The average person consumes about ten grams of fibre daily, less than half of the 30 grams recommended by most doctors and medical researchers.

There are two types of fibre: soluble and insoluble.

Soluble fibre, which includes pectin and plant gums, binds with bile in the intestine and is excreted in the faeces. Scientists believe that the liver compensates for the loss of bile by producing more bile salts in which cholesterol is a necessary ingredient. By reducing the amount of cholesterol circulating in the blood, soluble fibre helps to lower blood cholesterol levels.

Insoluble fibre contains compounds called cellulose and haemocellulose which absorb water and can improve the functioning of the large bowel. Insoluble fibre softens and bulks waste to help move it more quickly through the colon, thus helping to prevent constipation and reducing exposure to pesticides or naturally occurring carcinogens in food.

Good sources of soluble fibre include apple, oat bran, broccoli, carrots, dried peas and beans, potatoes, strawberries and other fruits and vegetables.

Good sources of insoluble fibre include celery, leafy green vegetables, whole grains, kidney and pinto beans, apples, and most other fruits and vegetables.

THE RIGHT AMOUNT I recommend 30–35 grams of fibre daily. In order to achieve this goal, you must be diligent about consuming daily at least five servings of fruit and vegetables daily and roughly six servings of whole grains (one slice of wholemeal bread or ½ cup of whole grain cereal = 1 serving.)

POSSIBLE BENEFITS

Cancer Fighter. In 1970 Dr Denis Burkitt published a study in which he noted that in countries where the population ate a diet high in fibre, cancer of colon and rectum was relatively rare. Other studies have confirmed the link between colon/rectal cancer and fibre. For example, a study at the Harvard School of Public Health recently examined the diets of 7,000 men. Researchers found that men who consumed the highest amount of saturated fat and the lowest amount of fibre were four times more likely to develop colon polyps, often a precursor to cancer.

Fibre may also offer protection against breast cancer. Studies have shown that women who develop breast cancer typically have higher levels of blood oestrogen than women who remain cancer free. A recent study sponsored by the American Health Foundation attempted to see if fibre could lower blood oestrogen levels. In the study, women were given 15 to 30 grams daily of wheat, corn or oat bran. At the end of two months, the women on the wheat bran experienced a dramatic drop in blood oestrogen levels, but not the women on the other forms of fibre.

Heart Disease. Several studies have shown that soluble fibre can lower blood cholesterol levels, which decreases the risk of coronary artery disease and stroke. For example, psyllium, derived from the ground-up husks of the psyllium plant, is used as a laxative and in cereal as a cholesterol-lowering agent. According to one study performed at the University of Kentucky Medical Service, a diet rich in psyllium flake cereal can reduce blood cholesterol levels by 12 per cent. Based on this study, psyllium appears to be especially effective in lowering LDL or so-called 'bad' cholesterol. (Psyllium may, however, cause an allergic reaction in some people.)

Oat bran is another popular cholesterol buster. Studies show that by eating roughly 20 g of instant oatmeal daily, you can cut your total cholesterol level by about six points, thus reducing your risk of heart attack by about 12 per cent.

Dried beans are also potent cholesterol cutters. A recent study showed that by eating 100 g of cooked beans daily, people with cholesterol levels of over 200 mg/dl can reduce their total cholesterol by as much as 20 per cent.

Gastrointestinal Disorders. Insoluble fibre can help to ward off the kinds of gastrointestinal ailments that plague middle age and beyond. First, it can prevent constipation—infrequent bowel movements or hard stool which is difficult to pass. Constipation is not just uncomfortable but can promote haemorrhoids, varicose veins in the area of the anus and rectum. People with a chronic history of constipation are also more likely to develop diverticular disease (diverticulosis and diverticulitis) which affects more than one-third of all adults over 50. Diverticulosis is characterised by the presence of saclike herniations (called diverticula) which can form in any part of the gastrointestinal tract, but more often than not in the colon. Symptoms of diverticulosis may vary from no symptoms at all to cramps, constipation or diarrhoea. Diverticulosis can develop into a more serious condition, diverticulitis, if the diverticula become inflamed. Diverticulosis is quite common among older people, and is usually treated with a high fibre diet. (Diverticulitis is treated with antibiotics and a low fibre diet.)

CAUTION If you are adding fibre to your diet, introduce it gradually. If you gobble up too much fibre too quickly you may develop wind and cramps. Drinking six to eight glasses of water daily will help relieve wind.

If you have any rectal bleeding or blood in your stool, contact your doctor immediately.

FLAX

FACTS As far back as 8,500 years ago, flax was a normal part of a diet that included other wild cereal grasses such as barley. In modern times flax has been used primarily as a source of linen and linseed oil. Today, however, researchers at the American National Cancer Institute are exploring the potential anti-cancer properties of an edible form of flax seed, and if their expectations prove correct, flax may once again become a dietary mainstay.

THE RIGHT AMOUNT Linseed oil is available in capsules or liquid from health food shops. Take one to three capsules or one to three tablespoons (10–30 ml) daily. Ordinary flax can become rancid very quickly so use only products that contain stabilised flax.

POSSIBLE BENEFITS

Anti-cancer. Flax contains 27 anti-cancer compounds including fibre, pectin, tocopherol (vitamin E) and sitosterol. It is also an excellent source of lignans, which are converted in the gut into compounds similar in structure to natural oestrogens produced by the body. Lignans are believed to deactivate potent oestrogens that can cause tumours to grow; like other phyto-oestrogens, they bind to oestrogen receptor sites on cells in place of the more potent oestrogens. Studies have shown that people who consume diets rich in lignans have lower levels of cancer of the breast and colon.

FOLIC ACID

FACTS In recent years pregnant women have been urged to take 400 mcg of this B vitamin daily to prevent neural tube defects in their babies. But folic acid is not just for the very young—it's for people of all ages, especially those who want to live to a ripe old age.

Folic acid helps in the formation of red blood cells and in nucleic acids, RNA and DNA, the genetic material in the cells.

The word 'folic' is derived from the 'foliage' because the acid is found in dark green leafy vegetables such as spinach and broccoli. It is also found in dried beans, frozen orange juice, yeast, liver, sunflower seeds, wheat germ and fortified breakfast cereals.

THE RIGHT AMOUNT The RDA for folic acid is 400 mcg, roughly the amount in 500 g of boiled spinach or ½ cup of peanuts. (Do not exceed 800 mcg.) Women on average get only half this amount. Supplements of folic acid are sometimes supplied in B-complex formulas—100 mcg is the usual amount found in supplements.

POSSIBLE BENEFITS

Heart Disease. Folic acid may lower the risk of heart disease by helping to maintain normal levels of homocystine, an amino acid found in the body. In a recent study performed at Harvard Medical School, men with even a slightly elevated level of homocystine were three times more likely to have a heart attack than men with the lowest levels. Based on the study, when given a folic acid supplement, homocystine levels dripped back to normal in most cases. Researchers at Harvard say that patients who are believed to be at high risk of having a heart attack should have their homocystine levels checked. Here's my advice: even if you are not at high risk of having a heart attack, it makes good sense to eat a diet rich in folic acid.

Cancer Fighter. Researchers at Brigham and Women's Hospital in Boston have linked a diet low in folic acid to a change in DNA that may allow cancer-causing genes to be expressed. In their study of 26,000 men and women, those with the lowest intake of folic acid had the highest level of adenomas (precancerous tumours) of the colon or rectum. At Tufts University, researchers are studying whether very high doses of folate—about 20 times the current recommended level—can help prevent colon cancer in people with precancerous polyps.

Low levels of folic acid have also been linked to cervical cancer. Each year, 6,000 women die of cervical cancer in the United States. Cervical dysplasia—cell abnormalities that, if untreated, often lead to cancer—can be caused by an infection with the human pappillomavirus (HPV). Cigarette smoking, multiple sex partners and an early age of first intercourse are also believed to increase the risk of cervical cancer. In a recent study performed at the University of Alabama, 300 women with cervical dysplasia were compared with 170 healthy women. These women were interviewed about their lifestyle and eating habits. As part of the study, blood levels for certain vitamins were also checked. The results: women with the highest levels of folic acid had the lowest levels of cervical dysplasia, even if they were infected with HPV. The researchers concluded that folic acid may offer some protection against this potentially lethal virus.

FO-TI

FACTS   According to Chinese legend, this herb (known as *ho shou wu* in China) can help prevent hair from turning grey. Fo-ti is a favourite longevity herb among Chinese herbalists and although there is little evidence to prove that it can help maintain hair colour, recent studies show that it may offer real protection against heart disease.

THE RIGHT AMOUNT   Fo-ti is available in capsules from Chinese herbalists and larger health food shops. Take one capsule up to three times daily.

POSSIBLE BENEFITS

Heart Disease. Several Chinese studies have shown that fo-ti can lower blood cholesterol levels, thus helping to protect against heart attack. In addition, this herb contains flavonoidlike compounds that strengthen and dilate blood vessels, improving the flow of blood to the heart.

PERSONAL ADVICE   The Chinese have a mystical reverence for fo-ti. According to traditional folklore, the older the root, the more powerful its rejuvenating properties!

GAMMA LINOLENIC ACID

FACTS   Gamma linolenic acid (GLA) is a fatty acid that is extracted from the seeds of evening primrose or borage plants. For centuries herbalists have valued both plants for their medicinal properties. Today, gamma linolenic acid is marketed as evening primrose oil and can be found in most chemists' and health food shops. GLA is a very popular over-the-counter treatment in Europe and the United Kingdom for a wide range of ailments ranging from premenstrual syndrome (PMS) to skin rashes. Recent studies suggest that it may help prevent cardiovascular disease, provide relief for rheumatoid arthritis and may even be used one day as a cancer treatment.

THE RIGHT AMOUNT GLA is available in capsule form. Take 250 mg up to three times daily.

POSSIBLE BENEFITS

Reduces Inflammation. In a study reported in the 1 November, 1993 issue of *Annals of Internal Medicine,* researchers at the University of Pennsylvania's Graduate Hospital in Philadelphia gave capsules containing 1.4 grams of GLA daily to 19 people with rheumatoid arthritis, an autoimmune disorder character-ised by inflamed and painful joints. Eighteen other RA patients received a placebo. After six months, the group on the GLA showed less pain and fewer signs of inflammation than the patients taking the placebo. The research team did not find any adverse side affects associated with GLA. More studies need to be done to see if GLA is an effective treatment for RA.

Heart Disease. Several studies have shown that GLA may lower cholesterol levels in some people. In one Canadian study, patients taking 4 grams of evening primrose oil daily experi-enced a 31.5 per cent decline in cholesterol after three months. However, other studies have shown that GLA has only a small effect on lowering cholesterol.

In a study conducted at McMaster University in Hamilton, Canada, researchers tested GLA's ability to prevent blood clots. Rabbits were fed various fatty acids, including GLA, for a four-week period. The researchers found that GLA appears to inhibit platelets (blood cells involved in the formation of blood clots) from adhering to the walls of blood vessels. Thus, GLA may help to prevent blood clots, a major cause of heart attack and stroke.

Cancer Fighter. A recent study performed at Nazam's Institute of Medical Sciences in India has shown that GLA can selectively kill tumour cells. In a clinical trial, six patients with gliomas, a particular type of tumour, were given GLA. All the patients showed mild improvement. This does not mean that GLA is a cure for cancer, although one day it may prove to be an effective treatment in conjunction with other therapies against certain types of tumour.

GENISTEIN

FACTS Genistein is a hot 'new' anti-cancer compound that has actually been around for thousands of years although until recently nobody has noticed. It is a recently identified isoflavone found in soya and soya-based products. For decades scientists have been mystified by the much lower incidence of many different forms of cancer in Asia compared with the United States and Western Europe. (For example, the breast cancer rate in the United States is 22.4 per 100,000; in Japan it is six per 100,000.) Recent studies suggest that genistein could be a potent cancer fighter.

Good sources of genistein include whole soya beans, tofu (bean curd), soya flower, soya milk, and rehydrated vegetable protein which can be used in place of chopped meat in Mexican foods such as tacos and chilli. (Soy sauce does not contain genistein.)

THE RIGHT AMOUNT Eat one or two portions of soya foods per day (about 75 g).

POSSIBLE BENEFITS

Prevents cancer. Since 1987, several hundred papers have been published on genistein's role as a possible cancer fighter. In 1993, a German study published in the *Proceedings of the National Academy of Sciences* found that in test tube studies, genistein blocked a process called angiogenesis which is responsible for the growth of new blood vessels. The researchers speculate that genistein may indirectly prevent the growth of tumours by thwarting the formation of the new blood vessels that are necessary to nourish them. In other words, genistein literally starves little tumours before they can grow into bigger problems. The researchers go on to note that, in animal studies, soya products have inhibited the formation of mammary tumours and they logically conclude that genistein may be the compound protecting Japanese women from breast cancer.

Autopsies of Japanese men show that prostate cancer is as common among Japanese men as it is among American men, but the cancer seems to grow much more slowly—so slowly that many die without ever developing clinical disease. Until recently there was no explanation for this phenomenon. However, researchers now suspect that genistein is actually blocking the growth of these tumours. The Finnish researcher Herman Aldercreutz and his colleagues compared blood plasma levels of isoflavones in Japanese and Finnish men. The levels of isoflavones were more than 100 times higher among the Japanese men, with genistein occurring in the highest concentration of any other isoflavone. The researchers concluded, 'A life-long high concentration of isoflavonoids in plasma (Japanese children have as high a urinary excretion as adults) might explain why Japanese men have small latent carcinomas that seldom develop to clinical disease.' (*The Lancet*, 13 November, 1993.)

Researchers Greg Peterson and Stephen Barnes of the University of Alabama tested whether genistein could block the growth of non-oestrogen-dependent human breast cancer cells. In this study, they showed that genistein thwarted the growth of breast cancer *in vitro*, and that the presence of an oestrogen receptor was not necessary for isoflavones to inhibit tumour growth. This suggests that the protective effect of isoflavones may be due not to their effect on hormones, but rather to the particular ability of genistein to block cell growth.

Genistein holds great promise as a potential cancer protector. However, more studies need to be done before this can be confirmed.

Heart Disease. Genistein is believed to inhibit the action of enzymes that may promote cell growth and migration. Some researchers speculate that by blocking the action of these enzymes, genistein may also prevent the growth of cells that form plaque deposits in arteries, in much the same way that it may prevent the growth of tumours.

GINGER

FACTS Ginger root is one of the most widely used herbs in the world. In China, where it is highly regarded as a 'warming herb', it was mentioned in the famous *Shen Nong Herbal*, which dates back to 3000 BC. Ginger is also a major medicinal herb in Ayurvedic medicine, the Indian system of traditional medicine which is rapidly gaining popularity in the West. In the United States, the National Cancer Institute has included ginger in its Experimental Food Programme which is exploring the cancer preventive compounds in different foods.

Herbal healers in the West have long prescribed ginger as a treatment for nausea and morning sickness.

THE RIGHT AMOUNT   Fresh ginger is sold at supermarkets and greengrocers. It can be used in cooking, or made into a tea. Ginger capsules and teas are available from chemists and health food shops. Take one capsule up to three times daily, or drink one to two cups of ginger tea.

POSSIBLE BENEFITS

Cancer Fighter. Ginger has an abundance of a compound called geraniol which may be a potent cancer fighter. In a recent study, Dr Charles Ellson of the University of Wisconsin, Nutrition Science Department, found that a mere 0.1 per cent of geraniol increased the survival rate of rats with malignant tumours, and studies elsewhere have shown that geraniol can enhance the effectiveness of anticancer drugs. More studies are being done to determine whether it will have similar effects on people.

Heart Disease. Several studies have shown that ginger can prevent platelet aggregation—that is, it can prevent blood cells from sticking together and forming blood clots. If a clot lodges in an artery leading to the heart or the brain it can cause a heart attack or stroke. In one Indian study, 20 healthy male volunteers were fed 100 grams of butter daily, which significantly increased their rate of platelet aggregation. However, when ten of the men were given five grams of dry ginger divided in two doses with the fatty meal, the ginger appeared to inhibit the degree of platelet aggregation.

Migraine. A Danish study has shown that ginger may help prevent migraine headaches and could relieve some of the symptoms that go with them, such as pain and nausea. Studies show that ginger has anti-inflammatory activity, which could explain why it would work as a pain reliever.

GINKGO

FACTS Do you have difficulty remembering the names of people, even if you have just been introduced to them? Do you find yourself becoming more forgetful? Increasing forgetfulness is one of the most negative stereotypes of ageing, and the bad news is that there is some truth in it. A recent survey of nearly 15,000 adults over the age of 55 revealed that about three-quarters of them had some difficulty remembering things. The good news is that the leaf from an ancient tree may help to perk up your memory. Recent studies suggest that extract from the ginkgo leaf may help improve memory, maintain mental sharpness and provide many other life-extending benefits.

The ginkgo, which dates back to before the last ice age, is one of the hardiest trees known to man: some live as long as 4,000 years. Although the ginkgo kernel has been used in Oriental medicine for hundreds of years, it was only in the 1970s that European researchers began investigating the potential medicinal properties of the leaf. Today, ginkgo is one of the most commonly prescribed drugs in Europe, for a wide range of problems ranging from memory loss and tinnitus (ringing in the ears) to haemorrhoids and headaches.

Although ginkgo products are sold in health food shops, they may soon be used as a serious drug. In 1988, a chemist at Harvard synthesised a ginkgo compound called ginkgolide B which, among other things, is being tested as a potential drug for asthma and as an aid to help prevent the rejection of transplanted organs.

THE RIGHT AMOUNT Ginkgo, which is growing in popularity, is available in most health food shops and even some chemists'. I recommend a supplement containing a solution of ginkgo biloba in an 8:1 extract. Take 100 mg tablets two times daily. The effects of ginkgo are short-lived—the dose lasts for only a few hours. There is no known toxicity.

POSSIBLE BENEFITS

Memory Booster. There are several reasons why older adults may have difficulty remembering. Stress, lack of physical exercise, poor mental stimulation and even subtle vitamin deficiencies may impair cognitive function. However, there is also a natural slowing down in mental processes due to decreased levels of certain chemicals in the brain. Electrical impulses or messages from the brain are transmitted along nerve cells called neurons. Neurons have long tendrils called axons which overlap with another neuron. Neurons 'communicate' with each other via chemicals called neurotransmitters, notably dopamine and noradrenaline. As we age, there is a decreased production of neurotransmitters, resulting in reduced alertness and memory retention. Animal studies have shown that ginkgo increases the level of dopamine, which improves the body's ability to transmit information. Several human studies have shown that ginkgo can improve mental performance among elderly people who have shown deteriorating mental function. Studies of younger people suggest that high doses of ginkgo can improve short-term mental processes and in his book *Next Generation Herbal Medicine*, herbalist Dr Daniel Mowrey suggested that one day university students may use ginkgo to help them prepare for exams.

Improves Circulation. Studies also show that ginkgo improves the blood flow to the brain (and to other vital organs), providing the oxygen and nutrients that the brain needs to function at peak capacity. As we age, circulation is often impaired by plaque deposits in the arteries delivering blood to the brain and other organs. Ginkgo helps to dilate or relax arteries and veins, thus improving the flow of blood throughout the body.

Antioxidant. Ginkgo is rich in flavonoids, potent antioxidants that protect the body against free radicals or unstable molecules which can damage healthy cells. Heart disease, cancer and even arthritis are just some of the diseases believed to be caused or worsened by free radical damage.

Prevents Blood Clots. Studies show that ginkgo inhibits blood cells from sticking together, thus preventing the formation of clots that could lead to heart attack or stroke. (If a clot lodges in an artery leading to the heart, it can cause a heart attack; if it lodges in an artery leading to the brain, it can cause a stroke.)

PERSONAL ADVICE Try taking ginkgo supplements for haemorrhoids. Many people swear that it is one of the most effective agents for helping to control bleeding and itching due to irritated haemorrhoids.

GINSENG

FACTS Of all the substances listed in the anti-ageing 'Hot Hundred', ginseng may be the most widely used. For 5,000 years the Chinese have revered this herb as a cure-all for nearly every ailment, from impotence to heart disease, and as an overall antidote to the ravages of ageing. In recent years ginseng has been promoted in the West as a tonic and a rejuvenator, which has generated a great deal of interest in this herb. At last count there were more than 3,000 scientific studies that had been performed on ginseng, most of these done in the Far East or in the former Soviet Union, where ginseng (a home-grown variety) is routinely given to athletes to improve stamina and performance. Although more research needs to be done, there is strong evidence that ginseng has many positive effects on the body and the mind.

There are three different types of ginseng: Panax ginseng is grown in Korea; American ginseng (*Panax quinquefolius*) is grown in the United States. Siberian ginseng (*Eleutherococcus senticosus*), grown in Siberia, is actually not ginseng at all but a close relative that has similar affects. All forms of ginseng have similar properties, with some differences. Korean ginseng is considered the strongest form, while American ginseng is milder and is highly prized in the Far East.

THE RIGHT AMOUNT Ginseng comes in many forms including capsules, tablets, tea and powder. I recommend American or Siberian ginseng—some people may find panax ginseng too stimulating, especially at night. For capsules, take one up to three times daily. For tea, drink one cup daily. If you use powder, mix 5 to 10 grams in liquid daily. Excess use of ginseng can make some people very jittery, so do not exceed the recommended dose.

CAUTION   In rare cases ginseng, which has a mildly oestrogenic effect on the body, can cause vaginal bleeding in postmenopausal women. If this happens, be sure to tell your doctor that you are using ginseng since vaginal bleeding can be mistaken for a symptom of uterine cancer. Do not use ginseng if you have high blood pressure or an irregular heart beat.

Be sure to buy ginseng products from a reputable company. Ginseng is expensive, and unscrupulous distributors may try to pass off cheaper products as the genuine extract.

POSSIBLE BENEFITS

Stimulant. Oriental healers contend that ginseng improves mental performance, especially in older people, and animal studies confirm that it may improve the capacity to learn. For example, rats given ginseng were able to run through a maze faster to find a food reward than were untreated rats. Several human studies found that people taking ginseng made fewer mistakes and could even complete tasks faster than those not taking it. There are several theories as to why ginseng may have a positive effect on learning. Some researchers speculate that it may indirectly stimulate the production of stress hormones that can increase stamina and prevent fatigue. However, ginseng also contains choline—a chemical in the brain which is essential for learning and memory retention—and this may also help to perk up mental activity (see page 40). More studies are needed to determine ginseng's exact effect on mental functioning.

Antioxidant. Ginseng contains antioxidants, substances which prevent cellular damage due to oxidation, or to exposure to unstable molecules called free radicals. Free radicals are believed to be responsible for promoting mutations in cells that could lead to cancer, and may also play a role in heart disease by promoting the formation of LDL or 'bad' cholesterol.

Cancer Fighter. Researchers at Japan's Kanazawa University

71

found that unpurified saponins, compounds found in ginseng, inhibited the growth of cancer cells and actually converted diseased cells into normal cells.

Lowers Cholesterol. Japanese researchers found that rats which were fed a high cholesterol diet showed a drop in cholesterol and a rise in beneficial HDL or 'good' cholesterol after being fed ginseng.

Anti-stress. Soviet scientist Dr I. I. Brekhman first coined the term 'adaptogen' to describe ginseng. According to studies performed by Brekhman, ginseng helps the body to cope better with stress by normalising body functions. For example, if blood sugar levels drop too low, or blood pressure rises too high, Brekhman contends that ginseng somehow brings the body back to normal levels. Although the concept of an adaptogen may seem foreign to westerners who take medication only when they are sick, it is in keeping with traditional Chinese medicine, which used ginseng (and other herbs) as a tonic to maintain overall health.

Menopause Aid. Ginseng contains compounds that are similar in action to oestrogen, the female sex hormone. Many women use ginseng to help control some of the unpleasant side effects of menopause, such as hot flushes, which may occur when oestrogen levels decline. (Interestingly enough, in countries where ginseng is commonly used, such as China and Japan, menopause is not considered a 'medical problem', nor do postmenopausal women routinely take oestrogen supplements.)

PERSONAL ADVICE Take ginseng one hour before eating. Vitamin C can interfere with the absorption of ginseng, so if you take a C supplement, allow two hours before or after taking ginseng to do so.

GLUTATHIONE

FACTS I call glutathione the 'triple threat anti-ageing amino acid' because it is synthesised from three amino acids—L-Cysteine, L-Glutamic acid and glycine, all of which are found in fruits and vegetables. Glutathione is a potent antioxidant which is synthesised by our own body cells. Studies have shown that it may help protect against cancer, radiation poisoning and the detrimental effects of cigarette smoke and alcohol abuse. Glutathione is a popular supplement in Japan, the country with the longest life span in the world. Although many orthodox American scientists have dismissed gluthathione supplements as worthless, a recent study sponsored by the Human Nutrition Research Center on Aging at Tufts suggests that they may help keep an ageing immune system healthy.

THE RIGHT AMOUNT Glutathione is present in fruits and vegetables, but cooking can reduce its potency. I recommend taking 50 mg capsules, one to two times daily.

POSSIBLE BENEFITS

Immune Booster. Dr Simon N. Meydani, a well-known re-searcher in the field of nutrition, who discovered that vitamin E has a positive effect on the immune system of elderly people, carried out tests to discover whether glutathione would have a similar effect on ageing white blood cells in animals and humans. In both animal and human studies, he found that glutathione gave the immune system a much needed boost. It not only improved the blood cells' ability to produce substances that can help ward off infection, but it also reduced the amount of inflammatory substances produced by the cells. Interestingly enough, glutathione had a greater effect on the sluggish cells of older people than on younger ones. More research needs to be done before we can say that glutathione is a bona fide immune booster, but the preliminary evidence looks good.

Anti-inflammatory. Glutathione has been used as treatment for allergies and arthritis, both conditions which are caused by an inflammatory response in the body.

PERSONAL ADVICE Here's more evidence that when it comes to ageing well, the adage 'use it or lose it' takes on new importance. Studies suggest that exercise may increase the level of antioxidants such as glutathione in older people.

GREEN TEA

FACTS If there were an Olympic competition for longevity, the Japanese would be the world champions. They have a longer life span than any other nationality, even though they are heavy smokers. What's their secret? Some researchers in the United States and Japan are looking for the answer in a cup of tea—no, they are not reading tea leaves, they are reading some impressive studies that suggest that phytochemicals found in green tea may help fight against cancer and heart disease.

Green tea, derived from the tea plant, is a rich source of potentially beneficial compounds called catechins. As tea undergoes processing, it loses some of its precious catechins to oxidation, but green tea is only very lightly processed, thus retaining more of its catechins than the heavily processed dry, black tea that is sold in the West.

THE RIGHT AMOUNT Sip one or two cups of green tea daily. Real green tea is found in health food shops or oriental markets.

POSSIBLE BENEFITS

Cancer Fighter. Researchers at the American Health Foundation in New York exposed mice to nitrosamines, potent cancer-causing agents in cigarette smoke. One group of exposed mice was given green tea, the other was not. The results: there were 45 per cent fewer cases of lung cancer among the mice taking green tea. In other studies of lab mice, green tea helped to slow the rate of tumour growth in mice exposed to ultraviolet radiation.

Does this mean that green tea will work as well in humans? There is some evidence that it might. The cancer rate in central Japan is lower than anywhere else in the country, and by coincidence this is the area where green tea is produced and where the people drink more of the stuff than in any other part of Japan. More studies remain to be done before we shall know for sure whether or not green tea is a bona fide cancer protector, but meanwhile, drinking a cup or two of tea a day cannot hurt and may just help.

Cholesterol Buster. Animal studies show that green tea catechins can reduce cholesterol levels in laboratory rats fed a diet high in saturated fat and cholesterol. Human studies have shown that people who eat a high cholesterol diet (averaging three egg yolks in one meal) can maintain normal cholesterol levels by sipping green tea with their meals. I am not suggesting that it will work this well for everyone, or that you can eat a high fat diet so long as you wash it down with green tea. However, adding green tea to an already sensible diet may be a good way to keep cholesterol levels in check.

PERSONAL ADVICE   Coffee drinkers take note: On average, brewed tea contains half the caffeine found in coffee, and is probably twice as good for you.

HAWTHORN

FACTS   Heart disease is a major killer in Western countries, which is why I believe this 'heart-healthy' herb will become very hot as the baby boom generation reaches middle age and beyond.

Since the 1700s, European herbalists have used preparations made from the hawthorn plant as a tonic for the heart. Today this herb is widely used throughout Europe, notably in France, Britain, Russia and Germany, and is gaining in popularity in the United States.

THE RIGHT AMOUNT   Hawthorn is available from herbalists and health food shops, both in capsule form or as a tea. Take one capsule up to three times daily. Drink one to three cups of tea daily.

CAUTION   If you are on any medication for your heart, do not discontinue or alter your dose without consulting your doctor or healer.

POSSIBLE BENEFITS

Heart Disease. Hawthorn is a well-researched herb, especially in Europe. Animal and human studies show that it has many positive effects on the cardiovascular system. Hawthorn is rich in bioflavonoids, compounds which strengthen capillaries, thus improving the flow of blood throughout the body. Studies on humans and dogs have shown that hawthorn can reduce blood pressure during exertion; animal studies also show that this herb can increase the contractility of the heart muscle, strengthening the heart's ability to pump blood. Hawthorn is sometimes prescribed along with the drug digitalis to regulate the heartbeat, as this reduces the required dose of digitalis. Other studies have shown that hawthorn may be useful as a treatment for angina (chest pain due to insufficient blood flow to the heart) and may also decrease the rate of heartbeat, preventing the heart from becoming overworked. Many natural healers believe that hawthorn can keep an ageing heart pumping like a young one!

HORSETAIL

FACTS Horsetail is a bamboolike marsh-dwelling plant which has been used for hundreds of years by herbalists as a treatment for rheumatoid arthritis. The herb is also a mild diuretic and is used by homoeopathic doctors as a remedy for urinary problems and enlarged prostate. There is a growing interest in herbs such as horsetail these days, due to the ageing population and the rise in age-related ailments such as arthritis and prostate problems.

THE RIGHT AMOUNT Horsetail is available in tablets or capsules at health food shops. Take up to three tablets or capsules daily. Some studies show that very high doses of the plant have been toxic to livestock, but the low doses recommended here should not have any adverse affects.

POSSIBLE BENEFITS

Rheumatoid Arthritis. Gold shots are sometimes used as a remedy for rheumatoid arthritis. Horsetail has been shown to absorb minute quantities of gold dissolved in water, and some herbalists believe that the gold residue in horsetail may be the reason why some people find it effective against the joint pain and stiffness associated with arthritis.

Hair Enhancer. According to the *Handbook of Medicinal Herbs*, the Meskawki Indians fed horsetail to their ponies to improve the floss of their hair. Horsetail is rich in silica, a mineral that is reputed to add shine and strength to hair and which is used in many shampoos and conditioners. Silica is also used to strengthen nails.

L-ARGININE

FACTS L-arginine is a non-essential amino acid—since the body produces it on its own, we do not need to get it in food. However, recent studies suggest that it may play an important role in maintaining health.

L-arginine can stimulate the growth and release of growth hormone, which is produced by the pituitary gland. As we age, the level of growth hormone steadily decreases, and some experts believe that the decline in L-arginine production may be responsible for many of the degenerative processes associated with ageing.

Good food sources of L-arginine include nuts, sunflower and sesame seeds, chocolate, raisins and brown rice.

THE RIGHT AMOUNT L-arginine is available in tablets and powder. Take 2000 mg daily at bedtime, about two hours after eating. L-arginine is often taken in combination with two other amino acids, 2000 mg ornithine and 1000 mg lysine.

CAUTION Do not give L-arginine to children or to adults with schizophrenia. L-arginine is reputed to promote herpes, so people with herpes should not use it. Very high dosages can cause deformities of the bones and enlarged joints.

POSSIBLE BENEFITS

Wound Healing. Many studies have demonstrated that L-arginine supplements can promote wound healing of burns and wounds after trauma such as surgery or injury. If you have been injured recently, or have undergone surgery, talk to your doctor or healer about taking an L-arginine supplement.

Cancer Fighter. Several studies have confirmed L-arginine's ability to inhibit the growth of tumours in animals. Studies involving human blood cells show that L-arginine increased the production of natural killer cells (important immune cells) and other compounds which can thwart the growth of tumours.

Male Infertility. Male seminal fluid contains as much as 50 per cent L-arginine. Several studies have linked a low sperm count to low levels of this important amino acid.

L-CARNITINE

FACTS If you are at risk of developing coronary artery disease, here is a potential life extender that you should know about. L-carnitine is a non-protein amino acid that is found in heart and skeletal muscle. Its primary job is to carry activated fatty acids across the mitochondria—the so-called 'powerhouse' of the cell—providing heart and skeletal cells with energy.

L-carnitine is widely used in Japan as a treatment for heart disease and is very popular in the United Kingdom. Enthusiasts claim that it can protect against heart disease and can improve physical stamina and endurance during exercise.

Severe L-carnitine deficiency is fairly rare and is associated with muscle weakness and cramps after exercise. People with kidney disease, severe infection, liver disease and other medical problems may develop L-carnitine deficiency. Some researchers believe that subtle forms of L-carnitine deficiency, which may go unnoticed, may increase the risk of having a heart attack.

Red meat—beef and lamb—and dairy products are the best natural sources of L-carnitine. Unfortunately, these foods are also high in saturated fat, which can promote heart disease. Therefore an L-carnitine supplement may be preferable to increasing your intake of meat.

THE RIGHT AMOUNT There is no RDA for L-carnitine. It is available in capsule form from health food shops. Take two

500 mg capsules daily. In rare cases, people taking over 1 gram of carnitine per day may develop a fishy odour which is caused by the breakdown of carnitine by intestinal bacteria. The odour usually disappears when the dose is cut back, but if it is troublesome you may want to discontinue use.

CAUTION   There are two kinds of carnitine—L-carnitine and D-carnitine. Some studies suggest that D-carnitine may be toxic, so stick to products containing only L-carnitine. If you have a heart condition, do not take this or any other drug without first consulting your doctor. In high doses (over 3 grams per day) L-carnitine may cause cramps or diarrhoea.

POSSIBLE BENEFITS

Heart Disease. Ischaemia is the reduction in the oxygen supply to the heart usually caused by the narrowing of a coronary artery, often due to atherosclerotic deposits or an arterial spasm. Several studies show that ischaemia can result in a reduction in carnitine in heart muscle. L-carnitine supplements appear to raise carnitine levels in heart patients, and increase their endurance. In one study involving 18 patients with coronary artery disease, exercise sessions were performed two weeks apart. Prior to exercise, one group of patients received carnitine, and the other received a placebo. Those on carnitine maintained lower blood pressure and were able to exercise longer and harder prior to experiencing angina or chest pain (a sign of ischaemia.) Other studies of heart patients have yielded similar results. We don't know for sure whether L-carnitine supplements can actually prevent ischaemia, but these studies suggest that they might.

In another study, 26 patients with high blood lipid levels were treated with 3 grams of oral L-carnitine per day. The result: a dramatic decline in total serum cholesterol and serum triglyceride. (Cholesterol levels over 200 mg/dl may increase your risk of having a heart attack. Triglyceride levels over 400 for men, and 190 for women are believed to increase the risk of heart disease.) In other studies, L-carnitine has been shown to raise HDL or 'good cholesterol'.

Improves Work-out. I have heard anecdotal evidence that

L-carnitine can improve stamina and strength during a work-out; however, there is no scientific evidence for this.

Alzheimer's Disease. The brain tissue of mammals is a rich source of carnitine. Some studies suggest that L-carnitine may be effective in slowing down the progression of Alzheimer's disease—for example, several European studies have reported that a daily supplement of L-carnitine (about 2 grams daily) can slow the mental deterioration typical of this disease. However, American researchers did not report good results from a major trial testing L-carnitine on Alzheimer's patients.

LEGUMES

FACTS Legumes (dried beans and peas) are a mainstay of many diets around the world. Rice and beans form a staple in Mexico, and *pasta e fagioli* (pasta and beans) are standard fare in Italy. Maybe not so coincidentally, people who live in countries where legumes are a major part of their cuisine have substantially lower rates of cancer and heart disease.

Legumes include all kinds of beans, ranging from kidney and haricot to lentils and black beans. All legumes are pretty much the same nutritionally, although there are some slight variations in fibre content and caloric value. Legumes are an excellent source of protein, although most lack certain essential amino acids that are found in meat (soya beans are the exception—they contain all eight essential amino acids that cannot be produced by the body). The amino acids that are missing in legumes are present in grains, so by eating legumes with a grain such as rice you can create a meal containing all eight essential amino acids.

THE RIGHT AMOUNT I recommend eating at least three legume-based meals weekly.

POSSIBLE BENEFITS

Cancer Fighter. Legumes contain many compounds that are believed to protect against cancer. They are a good source of *isoflavones*, compounds that block oestrogen receptors in some cells, and by doing so may deactivate potent forms of oestrogen that can trigger the growth of oestrogen-dependent tumour cells. About 30 per cent of all breast tumours are oestrogen-dependent.

Legumes are also rich in *protease inhibitors*, compounds that block the action of enzymes which can trigger cancer growth, and *phytic acid*, compounds which in animal studies have been shown to thwart the growth of tumours.

Legumes are an excellent source of *fibre*, substances in plants that are not digested and absorbed by the body. A diet high in fibre is believed to protect against some forms of cancer, particularly cancer of the colon. No one knows exactly how fibre helps to prevent cancer, but one theory is that it moves food more quickly through the colon. As food is broken down into its basic components, potential carcinogens are released into the gut. Some carcinogens may be naturally occurring; some may be from insecticides or added in processing. If food is speeded through the gastrointestinal tract, there is less exposure to these potential cancer threats.

Lowers Cholesterol. A study at the University of Kentucky showed that legumes are powerful cholesterol busters. Eating 100 g of cooked beans daily can in time reduce cholesterol levels of over 200 mg/dl by as much as 20 per cent.

Diabetes. As we age, we are much more likely to develop insulin resistance—that is, the body becomes less efficient at metabolising or utilising glucose (blood sugar). High levels of blood sugar are associated with diabetes, which increases the risk of heart attack, stroke and other vascular problems. Many researchers believe that diet may help to prevent diabetes, or at least delay its onset in some people. In particular, foods that avoid a heavy concentration of sugar in the bloodstream at one time may be better than foods that force insulin to work overtime. Complex carbohydrates, the kind found in legumes and grains, are just what the doctor ordered. They burn slowly and steadily in the body (not like sweets which burn very quickly), thus giving the insulin the time it needs to utilise glucose.

LEMONGRASS

FACTS   Lemongrass is one of many foods that are widely used in Asian cuisines but virtually nonexistent in Western cooking. Also known as citronella, lemongrass adds a fresh, lemony flavour to food. It is not only delicious, but studies show that lemongrass oil may help protect against heart disease by lowering cholesterol.

Fresh lemongrass and lemongrass oil are sold in specialist Asian shops and in health food shops. If using the whole plant, the lower part of the stalk is crushed and finely chopped. Lemongrass oil is used as a flavouring.

THE RIGHT AMOUNT   Use the plant or the oil in cooking whenever you can. Add one stalk of chopped lemongrass to stir-fry vegetables and other Asian dishes. Many recipes from the Far East call for lemongrass oil.

POSSIBLE BENEFITS

Heart Disease. Researchers at the University of Wisconsin gave men with high cholesterol 140 mg of lemongrass oil daily for three months. At the end of the study, 30 per cent of the men experienced a ten per cent decrease in cholesterol. The researchers suspect that a compound in lemongrass decreases the synthesis of cholesterol from fats.

LIGNANS

FACTS   People who live in countries such as in Asia and Africa, where plant food is a mainstay of the diet, have a much lower rate of many forms of cancer than people who live in Western countries where the diet is heavy in meat and light on fruits and vegetables.

For several decades researchers have been attempting to isolate the specific components in plant food which may help to prevent certain diseases. Scientists have studied various vitamins, minerals and fibre, the non-digestible food substance in plants that is not digested by the body. Each of these substances may play a role, but some may play a greater role than others. In 1979 a compound in fibre called lignan was discovered, and today, many researchers believe that lignans may be responsible for much of fibre's protective effect.

Many studies have shown that lignans have anticarcinogenic, antiviral and antifungal properties. They are also rich in phyto-oestrogens, hormone-like compounds which mimic the behaviour of natural hormones in the body.

Flaxseed is the best plant source of lignans, although wheat bran and rye also have these compounds. Smaller amounts can be found in many plants and vegetables.

THE RIGHT AMOUNT   Research on lignans is relatively new, so we have no idea of the precise amount needed to prevent cancer. I recommend eating foods that are rich in lignans, such as grains, fruits and vegetables. Bread made from flax is a particularly good source. If your health food shop does not sell this, you may be able to obtain the flax to add to your own homemade bread.

POSSIBLE BENEFITS

Cancer Fighter. There are several theories on why lignans may protect against cancer. Studies have shown that vegetarian and semi-vegetarian women have a much lower rate of breast cancer than women who eat meat. Researchers have measured the amount of lignans and oestrogen in the urine of vegetarian women, and have found that their urine contained higher amounts of both than did the urine of women who were not vegetarians. What was even more interesting was the fact that women who had breast cancer excreted much smaller amounts of lignans and oestrogen in their urine than either vegetarians or meat eaters, and had higher blood levels of oestrogen. From these studies, researchers suspected that lignans had a protective effect against breast cancer.

Other studies have shown that in the body lignans are converted into oestrogen-like compounds which mimic the behaviour of oestrogen. Some forms of naturally produced

83

oestrogen are believed to promote the growth of oestrogen-sensitive tumours. Certain cells in the body have receptors which bind with oestrogen and lignans, which are chemically similar to oestrogen, may compete with the more potent natural forms of oestrogen for space on oestrogen-sensitive cells. If natural oestrogen has no place to bind, it becomes deactivated, thus losing its ability to promote the growth of tumours. Excess oestrogen is excreted in urine.

Some researchers believe that lignans may also be protective against cancer of the prostate and colon.

LIGUSTICUM

FACTS Ligusticum (licidum or wallichii) is an important Chinese herb that is in hot demand in the West because of its reputation as an immune booster. This herb, combined with astragalus, reishi and other immune herbs, is used by natural healers to strengthen compromised immune systems (as in the case of AIDS patients or cancer patients receiving chemotherapy.)

Ligusticum is a highly revered herb in China, and is used in a famous woman's tonic, called 'Four Things Soup', which includes Dong Quai (see page 53).

There are more than 60 species of ligusticum throughout the world. In the Southwestern United States, Native Americans have long used *Ligusticum porteri* to treat viral, fungal and respiratory infections. You may find ligusticum marketed as Osha.

THE RIGHT AMOUNT Osha and ligusticum are sold in capsules and extract in health food shops. Take two to three capsules daily, or five to ten drops of extract in liquid two to three times daily.

POSSIBLE BENEFITS

Cancer Fighter. Many species of ligusticum have been shown to inhibit the growth of tumours in animals.

Cardiovascular. A stroke can occur if the flow of blood to the brain is impaired in any way. There have been many studies investigating ligusticum and its role in the prevention of stroke. Several animal studies performed in China show that ligusticum can promote circulation to the brain and prevent the formation of blood clots. When a stroke was simulated in animal tests, ligusticum helped restore circulation to the brain, thus minimising brain damage. One Chinese study involving 158 patients with transient ischaemic attack (tiny strokes) showed that ligusticum was even more effective than aspirin in helping to disperse blood clots and improve blood flow to the brain.

In China ligusticum has also been used to treat angina, a condition which is caused by a reduction in blood flow to the heart.

LIQUORICE

FACTS   When Westerners think of liquorice, they think of the liquorice-flavoured sweet that contains little if any of the real herb. In China, however, liquorice is the most widely used of all medicinal herbs. Five thousand years ago, liquorice was immortalised in the Shen Nong famous herbal and today it is highly regarded as a tonic and longevity herb. Recently, liquorice's potential health benefits have attracted the attention of Western scientists: it is currently under investigation by the American National Cancer Institute for its possible anti-cancer properties.

THE RIGHT AMOUNT   Take one capsule up to three times daily.

CAUTION   Liquorice should not be used by people with high blood pressure.

POSSIBLE BENEFITS

Menopause. Liquorice is frequently used to treat symptoms of menopause. Liquorice contains a glycyrrhizin, a hormonelike compound that appears to help normalise hormone levels in women.

Anti-cancer. Animal studies show that glycrrhetinic acid (derived from glycyrrhizin) can block carcinogen-induced tumour growth. More studies are being done to determine if liquorice is an anti-cancer herb.

Arthritis. Due to its anti-inflammatory action, herbal healers prescribe liquorice to treat the swelling, aches and pains of arthritis.

Anti-ulcer. Carbendoxolane, a compound found in liquorice, has been used successfully to treat stomach ulcers.

LUTEIN

FACTS Lutein is a member of the carotenoid family, a group of 600 compounds occurring naturally in fruits and vegetables (of which beta-carotene is the most well known.) Carotenoids are believed to offer special protection against many different forms of cancer and recent studies suggest that lutein may also be a cancer fighter. Carotenoids provide fruits and vegetables with their orange, red and yellow colours, but they are also found in green leafy vegetables where they are hidden by the green colour of chlorophyll.

Good sources of lutein are spinach, greens, turnip and mustard, broccoli, green peas, celery and kale.

THE RIGHT AMOUNT There is no RDA for lutein, but I recommend eating one serving of a lutein-rich vegetable daily.

POSSIBLE BENEFITS

Cancer Fighter. A recent study of 1,200 people performed at the University of Hawaii found that people who ate foods high in lutein had a lower risk of lung cancer than those who ate lower levels of lutein. Researchers suspect that lutein's anti-cancer properties are due to its antioxidant action.

Population studies have linked a high intake of fruits and vegetables, which are rich in carotenoids, with a lower risk of cancers of the head, neck, lung, oesophagus and colon.

LYCOPENE

FACTS Lycopene, a member of the carotenoid family, is a potent antioxidant that may prove to be one of the most important of all the phytochemicals.

Lycopene, which gives fruits and vegetables a reddish colour, is found primarily in tomato, ruby red grapefruit and red peppers.

THE RIGHT AMOUNT Eat one lycopene-rich food daily. Lycopene (along with other phytochemicals) is now available in capsule form. However, the studies linking lycopene to a reduced risk of certain forms of cancer have all been done on food, not on supplements. Therefore I still recommend getting your lycopene from food if you can.

POSSIBLE BENEFITS

Cancer Fighter. A few studies have linked low blood serum levels of lycopene to an increased risk of certain forms of cancer. No one is certain how lycopene may offer protection against cancer, but most researchers believe that its antioxidant properties may play a role.

- A study at the School of Public Health and the University of Illinois at Chicago showed a link between lycopene blood levels and cervical dysplasia, a precancerous condition in women.
- Bladder cancer is the most common malignant tumour of the urinary tract, and is prevalent among those aged 50–70. Recent studies have shown a link between low blood levels of lycopene and an increased risk of bladder cancer.
- Pancreatic cancer, one of the most lethal forms of cancer, primarily affects people between the ages of 50 and 80 and the disease is very difficult to treat. Researchers speculate that lycopene may offer some protection against pancreatic cancer, based on a recent study that showed that people with the lowest levels of lycopene had the greatest risk of developing pancreatic tumours.

MAGNESIUM

FACTS   As minerals go, magnesium is hardly a superstar—few people think about whether or not they are getting enough magnesium in the course of a day. And yet, as we age, magnesium may prove to be one of the most important minerals.

Magnesium is essential for calcium and vitamin C metabolism, and it also plays a role in the metabolism of phosphorus, sodium and potassium. This mineral is important for converting blood sugar into energy, and is necessary for effective nerve and muscle functioning.

In recent years magnesium has been touted as an essential mineral for heart health, and recent studies suggest that it may also play a role in helping to prevent diabetes, especially later in life.

Good sources of magnesium include nuts, unmilled grains, seeds, apricot, dried mustard, curry powder, dark leafy vegetables and bananas.

THE RIGHT AMOUNT   The RDA is 200–500 mg for adults. Magnesium is available in most multivitamin and mineral supplements and can also be purchased in the form of magnesium oxide or chelated magnesium supplements.

Magnesium and calcium supplements (with half as much magnesium as calcium) are an excellent source of both minerals.

People who drink heavily require extra magnesium.

CAUTION   Excess magnesium (over 1000 mg daily) can cause diarrhoea. Over time it can be toxic. Do not take a magnesium supplement if you have kidney disease.

POSSIBLE BENEFITS

Heart Disease. Epidemiological studies show that people who live in regions with high levels of magnesium in the soil and water have a lower rate of heart disease than the general population. Many other studies have shown that people who have heart attacks have a lower than normal level of magnesium in their body tissues. As far back as the 1950s, animal studies showed that high doses of magnesium can actually reverse atherosclerotic plaques. Other studies show that magnesium decreases blood pressure and improves the flow of blood to the heart. It is logical to conclude that magnesium plays some role in protecting against heart disease, although the precise role is not known. Some researchers, however, believe that magnesium works in conjunction with calcium to prevent fatal arrhythmias, in a similar way to calcium channel blockers.

In many hospitals, intravenous magnesium is routinely given to patients after they have a heart attack. The effectiveness of this treatment is still under debate, but several studies have shown that people who get intravenous magnesium after a heart attack have a significantly better survival rate than those who do not. However, a major American study involving thousands of heart attack patients did not support these findings.

Improves Glucose Handling. As people age they are likely to develop insulin resistance—that is, they cannot use insulin efficiently to turn glucose into energy; thus blood glucose levels rise, which can lead to diabetes. According to a recent study at the University of Naples, magnesium supplements can improve glucose handling in older people with insulin resistance. Other studies have shown that magnesium supplements can reduce blood pressure, and lower the risk of complications in patients who already have diabetes.

MELATONIN

FACTS Melatonin is a hormone secreted by the pineal gland in the brain during sleep. It is vital for the maintenance of normal body rhythms, especially the sleep-wake cycle, and appears to play a critical role in many other body functions. When I am travelling, I use melatonin to help ease the symptoms of jet lag, when normal sleep patterns are disturbed by a disruption in the daylight–darkness pattern. Melatonin helps to normalise the body's circadian rhythm which regulates sleep–wake cycles. Recently, it has been successfully tested as a cure for insomnia.

The production of melatonin declines dramatically with age.

Thousands of years ago, the ancient Greeks believed that melatonin was the 'seat of the soul'; today, many researchers suspect that it may be a natural anti-ageing hormone.

THE RIGHT AMOUNT   Synthetic forms of melatonin are sold in some health food shops in tablet or capsule form in 3mg strength. A faster acting sublingual tablet, which is placed under the tongue, is also available. Take one to three tablets or capsules (up to 9mg) about one and a half hours before bedtime. If using the sublingual form, take them 45 minutes before going to sleep. Occasional use preferred.

POSSIBLE BENEFITS

Longevity. In 1987, Swiss scientists published a study showing that adding melatonin to the drinking water of mice during darkness prolonged the life span of the animals by 20 per cent (about six months longer than average.) The researchers speculated that melatonin might help reduce stress and improve the function of the immune system in animals and, perhaps, in humans. Other animal studies have shown that the removal of the pineal gland (which produces melatonin) can result in an acceleration of the ageing process. In a review article published in the *International Journal of Neuroscience* (1990, Vol. 52, pp. 85–92), psychiatrist Reuven Sandyk, of the Department of Psychiatry of Albert Einstein College of Medicine in New York, stated, 'There is evidence from both experimental animal and human studies to suggest that decreased melatonin functions may accelerate the ageing process and thus support the notion that melatonin may function as an anti-ageing hormone.'

Some researchers speculate that melatonin be an antioxidant—that is, it prevents cellular damage associated with ageing by thwarting the action of free radicals. Others feel that melatonin may slow down ageing by controlling the timing of the release of certain hormones, proteins and neurotransmitters (chemicals that help nerve cells communicate with each other.)

Insomnia. Disruption in sleep cycles is a common ailment among older people, and many scientists have suggested that a reduction in melatonin may be responsible. In fact, recent studies show that melatonin may be a potent sleep aid. Researchers at Massachusetts Institute of Technology have found that melatonin can induce sleep in young volunteers within five or six minutes. Volunteers given a placebo took 15 minutes or more to fall asleep. In addition, those taking the melatonin slept twice as long as those taking the placebo. Scientists hope that melatonin may prove to be a safe, non-addictive sleep agent.

Breast Cancer. Several studies have linked a higher rate of breast cancer to both women and men who are in professions where they are exposed to low frequency electronic magnetic fields (EMFs). Researchers were puzzled by this finding and were not certain how or even if EMFs played a role in cancer. However, one recent study showed that exposure to EMFs can reduce the pineal gland's ability to produce melatonin at night, and some researchers now suspect that low blood levels of melatonin may trigger the growth of breast cancer cells. Although these findings are interesting, scientists still caution that the case of EMFs and melatonin is far from closed. Much more research is needed.

MENADIONE (VITAMIN K)

FACTS   When *The Vitamin Bible* was first published in 1979, little was known about menadione, also called vitamin K, except that it was essential for the synthesis of proteins involved in proper blood clotting. Nearly twenty years later, however, vitamin K is attracting the attention of researchers worldwide because of the possible role it may play in helping to prevent osteoporosis. At the USDA Human Nutrition Research Center at Tufts University there is a special laboratory devoted to investigating the relationship between vitamin K and ageing.

Vitamin K is formed by natural bacteria in the intestines. It is also found in green leafy vegetables, alfalfa, egg yolk, safflower oil, soya bean oil, kelp (seaweed) and fish liver oils.

THE RIGHT AMOUNT   The RDA for vitamin K is 100 to 250 mcg daily. I recommend taking a supplement of 50–100 mcg daily. Do not exceed 500 mcg daily. According to researchers at Tufts, older people may require higher levels of vitamin K due to a decreased rate of absorption.

People on long-term antibiotic regimens may develop a vitamin K deficiency.

CAUTION People taking blood thinners should not take vitamin K unless under the supervision of a doctor.

POSSIBLE BENEFITS

Osteoporosis. Several studies have shown that vitamin K supplements may help reduce the loss of calcium in urine, which contributes to the thinning of bones. For example, in one Dutch study presented at the New York Academy of Sciences special meeting on vitamins in 1991, researchers noted that a vitamin K supplement reduced urinary excretion of calcium in post-menopausal women, and was particularly effective in stemming the loss of calcium among those with a tendency to quick loss of calcium. Previous studies have linked a low level of vitamin K to an increased risk of fractures.

MILK THISTLE

FACTS Milk thistle preparations are popping up in health food shops everywhere and are already extremely popular. Since ancient times, the seeds from this weed have been used to treat many different ailments including digestive disorders. However, today's milk thistle is fast becoming known as the 'liver herb'.

Milk thistle contains silymarin, compounds which are members of the flavonoid family. Flavonoids are antioxidants and help protect cells from free radicals, unstable oxygen molecules which can cause dangerous mutations.

THE RIGHT AMOUNT Milk thistle is available in capsules. Take 175 mg three times daily.

POSSIBLE BENEFITS

Liver Disease. The liver is the most complicated organ in the human body. It performs many vital tasks including the production of bile, which is necessary for the breakdown of fat and the storage of glycogen to fuel the muscles. The liver also produces other important substances such as clotting factors (so that we don't bleed to death), blood proteins and more than a thousand different enzymes. One of the liver's most critical roles is the detoxification of drugs and poisons (such as alcohol) which may be taken externally or produced internally. Injury to the liver can be life-threatening. Inflammation of the liver is called hepatitis, and can be caused by drug toxicity or viral infection.

Many studies have shown that milk thistle has a strong therapeutic effect on the liver, protecting it from damage inflicted by toxins and disease. In fact, in Europe, milk thistle has been used as an effective treatment for viral hepatitis and cirrhosis of the liver (a condition caused by alcohol abuse). Many people take milk thistle daily as a 'liver tonic' to strengthen and protect this important organ.

MONOUNSATURATED FAT

FACTS Fat has become a dirty word lately, especially for people who are concerned about health and longevity, but eating monounsaturated fat may actually help you live longer. Studies show that in countries such as Italy and Greece, where the diet is rich in monounsaturated fat (mainly olive oil) the incidence of heart disease is a fraction of what it is in Britain and the United States.

There are three kinds of fats: saturated, polyunsaturated and monounsaturated. The degree of saturation is determined by the number of hydrogen molecules: the more hydrogen molecules, the more saturated the fat. Saturated fat is believed to promote the formation of plaque, which can lead to atherosclerosis.

Olive, canola (from rape seed) and avocado oil are excellent sources of monounsaturated fat. Nuts such as almonds, peanuts and walnuts are also rich in monounsaturates.

THE RIGHT AMOUNT I believe that people should consume no more than 20 per cent of their daily calories in the form of fat of any kind. (The late Nathan Pritikin and Dr Dean Ornish recommend no more than ten per cent, which I feel may be too difficult to adhere to.) Therefore, it is important to watch fat intake, even if it is 'good' fat.

Use 1–2 tablespoons of olive or canola oil in your salad or cooking daily.

If you eat nuts, keep the portions small.

POSSIBLE BENEFITS

Heart-Healthy. Although monounsaturated oil does not necessarily lower total blood cholesterol levels, it does raise the levels of 'good' HDL cholesterol. High levels of HDL are associated with lower rates of heart disease.

Recently, Israeli researchers found that olive oil was less prone to oxidative damage than polyunsaturated oil. Oxidative damage of blood lipids is believed to be a major cause of atherosclerotic lesions that can lead to a heart attack or stroke. Olive oil in particular is also high in vitamin E, an antioxidant which helps prevent heart disease and cancer.

Diabetes. A handful of studies suggests that monounsaturated fat may be beneficial for diabetics.

Longevity. Other studies have linked consumption of monounsaturated foods—notably nuts—to a longer life span and a dramatically lower rate of heart attack. In fact, a major study of 26,000 members of the Seventh Day Adventist Church showed that those who ate almonds, peanuts and walnuts at least six times a week had an average life span of seven years longer than the general population.

PERSONAL ADVICE Keep in mind that fat in any form contains nine calories per gram (as compared to four calories per gram for carbohydrate and protein.) Beneficial though monounsaturated fats may be, a little goes a long way.

MOTHERWORT

FACTS   As its common name implies, motherwort has a long
tradition of being used to treat problems of the female reproductive system. The Latin name for motherwort is *Lenonurus
cardiaca* and as that name implies, motherwort is also known
as a heart-healthy herb.

Motherwort contains compounds which can cause uterine
contractions. For thousands of years it has been prescribed by
herbal healers to bring on delayed menstruation or to speed up
childbirth. However, today it is gaining popularity as a menopause aid.

THE RIGHT AMOUNT   Take 10–20 drops of motherwort in
liquid up to three times daily, or drink one cup of tea.

CAUTION   Do not use this herb during pregnancy.

POSSIBLE BENEFITS

Heart. Motherwort is a mild sedative. It helps control palpitations and rapid heartbeat due to anxiety. It also temporarily
lowers blood pressure. This herb is frequently used to treat
anxiety related to the physiological changes that can occur during menopause.

Bloating. During menopause women often retain water due to
hormonal swings. This herb is a mild diuretic that can help
relieve some of the discomfort due to bloating.

PERSONAL ADVICE   If you are experiencing rapid heartbeat
or palpitations, consult your doctor or natural healer. It could
be a sign of a more serious problem.

NIACIN (VITAMIN B₃)

FACTS   If you have high cholesterol, or have had a heart
attack, this vitamin could save your life.

Niacin works with two other B vitamins, thiamin and

riboflavin, in the metabolism of carbohydrates. It is also essential for providing energy for cell tissue growth. The body produces niacin from tryptophan, which is abundant in milk and eggs. Recent studies suggest that as people cut back on high fat and high cholesterol foods, such as milk and egg products, they may become deficient in niacin.

In recent years, niacin has gained fame as a potent cholesterol-lowering agent.

THE RIGHT AMOUNT   The RDA is 15–20 mg. High doses—the kind prescribed to cut cholesterol—can result in unpleasant side effects such as flushing and itching. If you are using niacin to lower cholesterol, I recommend the 'no flush' niacin supplements with inositol hexanicotinate. Supplements are available in 50 to 1000 mg doses in powder or pill form. Usually, between 800 mg to 1200 mg daily are needed to lower cholesterol. However, you can reduce the niacin dose by taking it with chromium picolinate—take 100 mg of niacin with 600 mg of chromium picolinate daily.

CAUTION   High levels of niacin can interfere with the control of uric acid, bringing on attacks of gout in people who are prone to this disease. Niacin may also interfere with the body's ability to dispose of glucose and may promote liver abnormalities. I therefore recommend using niacin only under the supervision of a doctor or natural healer. (Given the side effects of some of the other cholesterol-lowering drugs, however, niacin is relatively safe.)

POSSIBLE BENEFITS

Heart Disease. In 1975 the Coronary Drug Project, a major study, reported that niacin could dramatically reduce cholesterol levels and, even better, could cut the rate of second heart attacks by 30 per cent. A 15-year follow-up study comparing niacin to clofibrate, another cholesterol-lowering drug, found that even though both agents lowered cholesterol, patients who had taken the niacin had significantly fewer heart-related deaths than those who had taken the clofibrate.

Other studies confirm that niacin can lower both cholesterol and triglycerides, and can raise the level of HDL or 'good' cholesterol.

Cancer Fighter. There is some evidence that niacin may offer a measure of protection against cancer. In a recent study, scientists at the University of Kentucky's Markey Center tested the effect of niacin deficiency on human and animal cells. Cells that were deprived of niacin began to show signs of malignant changes that could lead to cancer. More studies need to be done on the role of niacin in cancer.

NITROSAMINE BLOCKERS

FACTS Nitrosamines are cancer-causing compounds that are formed during normal digestion. They can occur when nitrites, a commonly used food preservative, or nitrates, a naturally occurring chemical in food, combine with amino acids. Nitrosamines can destroy DNA, which may lead to cancerous changes in cells. Several years ago, researchers at Cornell University reported that certain foods, such as tomatoes, green peppers, strawberries, pineapples, and carrots, can help prevent the formation of these troublesome nitrosamines. Initially it was believed that vitamin C was the primary nitrosamine blocker in these foods, but in a recent article in the journal *Agriculture and Food Chemistry*, Cornell University food scientists reported the discovery of two other compounds in tomatoes—p-courmaric acid and chlorogenic acids—which appear to be potent nitrosamine blockers. This has led to the belief that there are probably other nitrosamine blockers in fruits and vegetables that have yet to be identified.

You cannot get these compounds in a pill or capsule—you must eat the fruit or vegetable. Cooking does not destroy the compounds and they are also present in juice.

THE RIGHT AMOUNT There is no RDA for nitrosamine blockers. Eat a wide variety of fruits and vegetables daily. I make a point of eating a tomato or drinking a glass of tomato juice every day.

POSSIBLE BENEFITS

Cancer Fighter. Researchers at Cornell University tested tomato juice on volunteers. After drinking the juice, the volunteers produced fewer cancer-causing nitrosamines. Although more studies need to be done, there is evidence that eating foods rich in nitrosamine blockers may help to prevent cancer.

PERSONAL ADVICE Nitrites are added to cured meats such as bacon to prevent botulism and as a colouring agent. Try to buy nitrite-free products, which are available at many supermarkets and delicatessens.

NUCLEIC ACIDS (DNA AND RNA)

FACTS DNA (deoxyribonucleic acid) and RNA (ribonucleic acid) are present in the nucleus of every cell in the body, and are essential for the production of new cells, cell repair and cell metabolism. As we age, cells begin to wear out and eventually die. While we are young we grow new cells very quickly, but as we age we replenish cells more slowly. Internally, our body systems begin to slow down and externally we begin to show signs of wear and tear. Some researchers believe that ageing may be a result of a decline in the level or effectiveness of these important nucleic acids. The theory goes that if we replenish the lost nucleic acids, we may be able to halt or even reverse the ageing process.

Good food sources of nucleic acids include Portuguese sardines (water packed), salmon, wheat germ, asparagus, mushrooms and spinach.

THE RIGHT AMOUNT Try to include some or all of the foods listed above in your weekly diet.

CAUTION Drink at least eight glasses of fluid daily if you are eating a diet rich in nucleic acids. RNA can raise uric acid levels which may trigger gout in susceptible people. If you have a tendency to develop gout, avoid foods that are high in nucleic acids.

POSSIBLE BENEFITS

Longevity. A handful of studies suggests that nucleic acids may increase the life span of animals. For example, in one study reported in the *Journal of the American Geriatrics Society* almost twenty years ago, five laboratory mice were given weekly injections of DNA and RNA, and five were untreated. The untreated mice died within 900 days, while the treated mice lived between 1,600 and 2,250 days. Researchers also noted that the mice given nucleic acid looked healthier and were more alert than the other mice. More studies need to be done to confirm whether nucleic acids are truly a 'fountain of youth'.

There is anecdotal evidence that nucleic acids may have a dramatic effect on humans. In his book *Nucleic Acid Therapy in Ageing and Degenerative Disease*, Dr Benjamin Frank reports on his experiences treating patients with nucleic acid therapy. Based on Dr Frank's observations, patients given nucleic acid supplements showed a marked improvement in the colour and texture of their skin, a reduction in age spots and an increase in energy level.

OAT BRAN

FACTS Oat bran contains a compound called beta-glucan, a potent cholesterol-lowering agent and a form of soluble fibre.

Good sources of oat bran include oat bran cereal and high fibre oatmeal. Instant oatmeal (the kind that cooks in the bowl) usually has less oat bran than ordinary oatmeal.

THE RIGHT AMOUNT A bowl of oatmeal and a couple of oatcakes daily can help reduce a high cholesterol, and keep a normal cholesterol in check.

POSSIBLE BENEFITS

Heart Disease. There have been numerous studies documenting oat bran's ability to lower cholesterol. When combined with a normal, low fat diet, about 50g of oats daily can reduce cholesterol by five to ten per cent. Oat bran can also lower LDLs, the 'bad cholesterol', and can raise HDLs, the 'good cholesterol'.

Diabetes. Researchers at the University of Kentucky have found that oat bran can help improve glucose and blood lipid levels in diabetics, helping them to reduce or eliminate their need for insulin.

OCTACOSANOL

FACTS   Octacosanol is a natural substance present in small amounts in many vegetable oils. A popular commercially marketed form of octacosanol is made from wheat germ oil. Proponents of octacosanol contend that it is a treasure trove of phytochemicals that can increase energy, improve oxygen utilisation and even prevent heart disease. Octacosanol is an excellent source of another member of the anti-ageing 'Hot Hundred'—vitamin E.

Good food sources of octacosanol include wheat germ, whole grains and alfalfa.

THE RIGHT AMOUNT   Supplements of 1000–6000 mcg per tablet are available at health food shops. Take one tablet daily.

POSSIBLE BENEFITS

Improves Stamina. Studies suggest that octacosanol may improve exercise performance in animals and humans. Octacosanol is believed to reduce oxygen debt—that is, it helps the body utilise oxygen more efficiently during times of stress. If you take octacosanol, you are therefore less likely to be huffing and puffing after a strenuous work-out.

Heart Disease. Octacosanol contains plant sterols, compounds which, in animal and human studies, have been shown to reduce cholesterol levels. However, the high vitamin E content of octacosanol may also play a role in reducing cholesterol by preventing the oxidation of LDL or 'bad' cholesterol which can lead to the clogging of important arteries.

OMEGA-3 FATTY ACID

FACTS   In the 1970s scientists noticed an interesting phenomenon: although Eskimos consumed gobs of fat daily, they had
an exceptionally low rate of heart disease and cancer. But unlike
typical American and British people who also ate lots of fat—
notably from meat and dairy products—the predominant fat in
the Eskimo diet was in the form of omega-3 fatty acid. Omega-3
is found primarily in marine plantlife called phytoplankton,
which are eaten by fatty fish, a mainstay of the Eskimo diet. On
land it is present in some plant food including flax seed and
purslane, a plant that is used in salads.

Since the 1970s there have been hundreds of studies performed worldwide on omega-3 fatty acid. These have shown
that omega-3 does indeed offer protection against heart disease
and possibly many other ailments.

Omega-3 contains two polyunsaturated fats: decosahaenioc
acid (DHA) and eicosapentaenoic acid (EPA).

Good food sources include fish such as salmon, mackerel,
albacore tuna, halibut and sardines.

THE RIGHT AMOUNT   According to the American National
Heart and Lung Institute, eating as little as 1 gram of omega-3
fatty acid daily may reduce the risk of cardiovascular disease by
as much as 40 per cent. Omega-3 fatty acid is available in capsule
form. Take three to six capsules daily.

Super EPA—a more concentrated form—is also available.
Take three capsules daily.

Flax seed oil capsules are another source of omega-3 fatty
acid. Take 1–2 capsules (1000 mg) daily with meals.

Fatty fish, however, is the best source—in fact, studies suggest
that the whole fish may be more effective than simply taking an
oil supplement. Include plenty of the fish mentioned above in
your diet.

CAUTION   Do not take omega-3 supplements without first
consulting with your doctor if you are already taking a blood
thinner or use aspirin daily. Excessive amounts of omega-3 fatty

acids may cause bleeding which can result in haemorrhagic stroke.

POSSIBLE BENEFITS

Heart Disease. Epidemiological studies document a lower rate of coronary artery disease among fish eaters, Greenland's Eskimo population and the Japanese.

Omega-3 fatty acid appears to have several positive effects on cardiovascular health. It is a blood thinner and may help prevent the formation of blood clots that can lead to a heart attack. A recent study of 15,000 people in four communities in the United States demonstrated that an increased intake of fatty fish can make a positive difference in terms of cardiovascular health. In this study, researchers compared the level of clotting factors (proteins found in the blood that can contribute to the formation of clots) to the amount of fatty fish in people's diet. Those who ate even one additional daily serving of fish had lower levels of three clotting factors that have been implicated in the development of coronary artery disease. Those with the highest levels of omega-3 fatty acid intake had higher levels of a fourth protein, protein C, a natural anticoagulant.

Several studies have shown that omega-3 fatty acid can lower total cholesterol and triglycerides in people who also cut back on saturated fat. In a Danish study, pathologists who autopsied fatty abdominal tissue and coronary arteries of 40 deceased people found a direct correlation between the amount of omega-3 fatty acid in the tissue and the degree of narrowing of the coronary arteries due to atherosclerosis. In other words, omega-3 fatty acid appears to prevent the formation of atherosclerotic plaque that can hamper the flow of blood to the heart.

A recent animal study performed at Australia's Commonwealth Scientific and Industrial Research Organisation in Adelaide investigated the effects of dietary fat on susceptibility to ventricular fibrillation, a potentially lethal heart arrhythmia. According to the study, animals who were fed fish oil were better able to withstand induced heart arrhythmias than those fed sunflower oil. The researchers concluded that omega-3 fatty acid may help prevent heart arrhythmias in humans.

Stroke. A long-term Dutch study shows that men who consumed more than 20g of fish per day had a lower risk of stroke than those who ate less fish. This is believed to be the first reported finding of a connection between higher fish consumption and lower stroke risk.

Cancer Fighter. In numerous animal studies, omega-3 fatty acid has delayed the onset of tumours and decreased the rate of growth, size and number of tumours in animals in which cancer was induced. Interestingly enough, in similar studies, other forms of fat typically increased tumour growth.

Arthritis. Omega-3 fatty acid has an anti-inflammatory action in the human body—that is, it alters the biological pathways that trigger inflammation, which is responsible for the pain and stiffness of arthritis and other related conditions. In several studies, patients with rheumatoid arthritis reported a decrease in symptoms after taking omega-3 fatty acid supplements in addition to their nonsteroid antirheumatic drugs.

Diabetes. In a Dutch study of 175 older people (64–87) over three years, those who ate fish were found to be least likely to develop glucose intolerance, a common problem among older adults, which can lead to diabetes.

PAPAIN

FACTS If you find yourself taking more and more antacids, you are not alone. As we age our digestive system becomes less efficient, and as a result, indigestion is a common malady among people over 50. Natural compounds such as papain, which is derived from papaya, may help to quiet an angry gut. Papain contains two enzymes, papain and prolase, which help to break down protein.

THE RIGHT AMOUNT Chewable papain supplements are sold in health food shops. Chew one to three tablets half an hour before eating.

POSSIBLE BENEFITS

Digestive Aid. In older people, indigestion is often due to the inability of the body to produce enough hydrochloric acid to break down food effectively. Although there has been little scientific research in this area, anecdotal evidence suggests that papain supplements may help improve digestion and reduce the need for antacids.

PERSONAL ADVICE If you are suffering from a great deal of wind or bloating, although it is probably simple indigestion, it could be a symptom of another underlying problem. Check with your doctor before trying self-medication.

PECTIN

FACTS Everyone has heard that 'an apple a day will keep the doctor away'. However, not everyone knows that pectin may be the reason why apples are so healthy. Pectin is a form of soluble fibre found in fruits and vegetables and recent studies suggest that it may be a potent force against both cancer and heart disease.

Good food sources of pectin include apple, banana, the pulpy portion of grapefruit, dried beans and root vegetables.

THE RIGHT AMOUNT Try to eat some pectin-rich foods daily. If you have high cholesterol, consider taking pectin capsules, which are available at most health food shops. (Take 1–2 capsules after each meal.) Pectin powder is also sold in health food shops: sprinkle 12g of pectin powder in your food. It has no flavour and adds body to yogurt, puddings or fruit salads.

POSSIBLE BENEFITS

Heart Disease. Several forms of pectin appear to lower blood cholesterol levels. Researchers at the University of Florida gave 27 people with high cholesterol either three tablespoons of powdered grapefruit pectin daily, or a placebo. After 16 weeks the group taking the pectin showed a 7.6 per cent reduction in cholesterol, and a 10.8 per cent reduction in LDL or 'bad' cholesterol. The group taking the placebo showed no change. Although powdered grapefruit pectin is more potent than plain grapefruit, eating one or two whole grapefruit daily—not just the segments but the pulpy portion between the segments—would probably also significantly lower cholesterol (in combination with a low fat diet).

Carrot, which contains calcium pectate, also appears to be a cholesterol buster. In fact, according to the USDA, eating two carrots a day may reduce total cholesterol levels by as much as 20 per cent.

Eating two apples a day may keep the cardiologist away. A recent study showed that people who ate two apples daily could reduce total cholesterol by as much as 16 per cent.

Cancer Fighter. Researchers at the University of Texas Health Science Center in San Antonio recently discovered that fibre may help to prevent colon cancer. The researchers fed laboratory rats a carcinogenic agent that predisposed them to develop colon cancer. One group of rats was fed a high pectin diet, the other group was fed a normal diet. After 24 weeks, the group on the high pectin diet had a significantly lower rate of colon cancer than those fed the normal diet. (In addition, the rats on the high pectin diet had a 30 per cent drop in cholesterol.) The pectin performed two roles: first, it increased the rate at which food passed through the gastrointestinal tract, which reduced the rats' exposure to carcinogens, and secondly, it bound with digestive bile, a derivative of cholesterol (thus reducing blood cholesterol levels.)

PHYTIC ACID

FACTS In the 1970s researcher Denis Burkit published a now famous study in which he showed that in Third World countries, where people ate a diet rich in plant foods, the rate of various forms of cancer was significantly lower than in the West. Dr Burkit attributed the reduced rate of cancer to a higher intake of fibre, and soon people throughout the Western world were stuffing themselves with bran and other sources of fibre. However, some researchers speculate that although fibre may be beneficial, the real hero may be phytic acid, a major ingredient in grains, nuts and legumes (dried beans such as soya beans and lentils).

Phytic acid is an antioxidant: it protects cells against oxidative damage from free radicals or unstable oxygen molecules, which can cause mutations in DNA. It is also a chelator, which means that it binds easily to metal, particularly iron. In the presence of oxygen, iron can create free radicals that attack DNA. Phytic acid can prevent this damage from occurring by binding with the iron, thus keeping it away from oxygen.

THE RIGHT AMOUNT There is no RDA for phytic acid. I recommend eating a diet rich in grains and legumes. Although nuts are an excellent source of phytic acid, they tend to be high in fat, so eat them sparingly.

POSSIBLE BENEFITS

Cancer Fighter. In several animal studies, phytic acid has been shown to inhibit the growth of tumours, especially in the colon. In one review of phytic acid published in *Free Radical Biology and Medicine* (Vol 8, 1990), researchers noted that in populations where people eat high quantities of red meat, which is rich in iron, 'the simultaneous presence of phytate may act to suppress iron-driven steps in carcinogenesis.'

POTASSIUM

FACTS High blood pressure, characterised by a systolic pressure over 140 and a diastolic pressure over 90, is a leading cause of heart attack and stroke. The older you are, the greater the risk of developing this potentially lethal disease. There is strong evidence, however, that dietary potassium intake may help to prevent high blood pressure, and may even be used to enhance the effect of antihypertensive medications.

Potassium is an essential mineral that assists in muscle contraction and works with sodium to maintain the fluid and electrolyte balance in body cells. Nerve and muscle function may suffer when the sodium/potassium balance is wrong. Potassium is also critical to maintaining a normal heartbeat, and in cases of severe potassium deficiency the heart can develop a dangerous arrhythmia or irregular beat.

Potassium is found in fruits and vegetables and dairy products. Good sources include banana, orange, cantaloupe, dried apricots, potatoes and plain low fat yogurt.

THE RIGHT AMOUNT The minimum daily requirement for adults has been estimated to be 2000 mg daily. Potassium is available in most high potency multivitamin and multimineral preparations. Excess amounts (over 18 grams) can be toxic. A banana contains 560 mg of potassium.

If you consume large quantities of coffee, are taking diuretics, have severe diarrhoea and/or vomiting, or have hypoglycaemia (low blood sugar) you may be deficient in this mineral. People on very low calorie weight loss diets may also have a potassium deficiency.

CAUTION People with kidney disease should not take a potassium supplement or consume foods high in potassium.

POSSIBLE BENEFITS

Lowers Blood Pressure. A recent Italian study, reported in the *Annals of Internal Medicine*, underlined the importance of eating a diet rich in potassium, especially if you have high blood pressure. Fifty-four patients with controlled hypertension were randomly assigned to one of two groups. One group was given advice aimed at increasing potassium intake through diet; those in the other group remained on their usual diet. Potassium intake among both groups was checked monthly by referring to the patients' food diaries and urinary potassium excretion. At the end of the year, the group on the high potassium diet found that they needed far less medicine to control their blood pressure than the group not eating potassium-rich foods. The researchers concluded, 'Increasing the dietary potassium intake from natural foods is a feasible and effective measure to reduce antihypertensive drug treatment.'

PERSONAL ADVICE If you are taking medication for high blood pressure, do not discontinue it, but work with your doctor to see if you can decrease your need for medication by increasing your potassium intake. Eating a banana and a baked potato daily can increase your potassium intake by 1200 mg.

PROPOLIS

FACTS Propolis is a by-product of honey. It is a resinous material made from leaf parts and tree bark, which is used by honeybees to cement together their hives. For thousands of years honey and its related products have been valued for their medicinal properties. Hippocrates used propolis to treat sores and ulcers and Nicholas Culpepper (1616–1654)—perhaps the most famous herbalist of all time—recommended it to be used externally on wounds. Modern herbalists use propolis to ease cold symptoms and soothe a sore throat, and recently scientists throughout the world have begun to recognise that this substance may not only be an effective treatment for minor ailments, but may help to prevent a very major one—cancer.

THE RIGHT AMOUNT Propolis is available in many different forms. Honey is a rich source, and pure propolis can be bought in capsule form at health food shops. Take 500 mg capsules three times daily.

Propolis salve may be used externally on sores. Propolis lozenges (which have a pleasant, sweet taste) are good for a sore throat.

POSSIBLE BENEFITS

Cancer Fighter. For decades, proponents of natural foods have touted propolis for its anti-cancer properties. Recently, serious researchers have investigated these claims. Scientists at the American Health Foundation in Valhalla, New York, tested caffeic acid esters, a compound found in propolis, for potential use against cancer. In the study, rats were fed a potent carcinogen and some of the rats were also fed caffeic acid esters from propolis. After nine weeks, the rats given the propolis compounds showed significantly less precancerous changes in colon cells than those not fed the propolis. Based on this and similar studies, it appears as if propolis can inhibit the growth of cancerous cells in the colon. Other studies are needed to determine whether it is useful against other forms of cancer.

Anti-inflammatory. Propolis may be similar to aspirin in that it blocks the enzymes that produce prostaglandins, natural hormone-like substances which can cause pain, fever and inflammation.

Anti-viral. Propolis is rich in bioflavonoids, substances which appear to help protect against viral invasion. Viruses are encased in a protective protein coat and researchers believe that the flavonoids in propolis may inhibit an enzyme in the body that strips viruses of their protective coating, thus allowing the infection to spread to other cells. As people age and their immune system weakens, propolis may give the immune system a much needed boost against common viruses which can cause colds and flu.

Prevents Gum Disease. Periodontal problems are common from middle age on. Very often, as people age, the gum line begins to recede, causing inflammation, bleeding and infection. This can lead to the weakening of the bone structure in the mouth, which can result in tooth loss. Some researchers believe that the flavonoids in propolis not only reduce inflammation, but also strengthen the blood vessels in the gums, making them less prone to injury.

PROTEASE INHIBITORS

FACTS Protease inhibitors are compounds that inhibit the action of certain enzymes which promote tumour growth. The American National Cancer Institute is investigating their potential anti-cancer properties.

Protease inhibitors are abundant in legumes (soya beans in particular and other dried beans) and whole grains.

THE RIGHT AMOUNT There is no RDA for protease inhibitors. I recommend eating at least one food daily that contains them.

POSSIBLE BENEFITS

Cancer Fighter. Several animal studies have shown that protease inhibitors can inhibit the growth of cancer. For example, soya beans contain a unique protease inhibitor—the Bowman–Birk Inhibitor (BBI), which has been shown to stop the spread of many different forms of cancer. In rats fed a carcinogen known to induce colon cancer, adding BBI concentrate to their diet suppressed the formation of tumours in 100 per cent of the animals. In another study of mice fed a carcinogen known to induce liver cancer, BBI suppressed the formation of tumours by 71 per cent. The NCI is now conducting human cancer prevention trials using BBI on people at high risk of developing cancer.

PSYLLIUM SEED

FACTS Ground psyllium seed is a popular cure for constipation, a problem which seems to be a common ailment among the older population. For years doctors have recommended psyllium as a natural way to regulate bowel function in people with digestive disorders such as irritable bowel syndrome and chronic constipation.

In addition, psyllium is a highly effective and safe cholesterol-lowering agent.

THE RIGHT AMOUNT I recommend a teaspoon to a tablespoon of psyllium daily in juice or water. Psyllium is sold in powder form in chemists' and health food shops and is the active ingredient in several over-the-counter medications. Some psyllium products contain other herbs, including slippery elm bark and acidophilus, which can help ease some of the wind and bloating that can occur when you first use psyllium. Ask at your local health food shop.

CAUTION In rare cases psyllium may cause allergic reactions in some sensitive individuals. If you are allergic, talk to your doctor before using psyllium. In addition, to prevent wind, drink 6–8 glasses of water daily.

POSSIBLE BENEFITS

Heart Disease. Several studies show that psyllium can lower blood cholesterol from high levels to safer levels. In one study, 26 men with cholesterol levels over 240 mg/dl were divided into two groups. (The range was 180 mg/dl to 314 mg/dl.) One group was given one packet of a psyllium product (3.4 g) three times daily in water before each meal. At the end of eight weeks, the average cholesterol level in the treatment group had dropped to 211 mg/dl. The level of LDL or 'bad' cholesterol had also dropped substantially.

In another study by fibre expert James W. Anderson of the University of Kentucky Medical Service, 44 people with elevated cholesterol levels were given either psyllium flake cereal or wheat bran flake cereal daily for six weeks. The results: the group eating the psyllium flake cereal had an average 12 per cent drop in cholesterol but the group eating the wheat bran had no change.

PYCNOGENOL

FACTS Pycnogenol is made from a patented blend of bioflavonoids found in fruits, vegetables and other plants. Widely used in Europe and the Far East, it is being touted as an anti-ageing supplement.

Pycnogenol was invented by Professor Jacques Masquelier of the University of Bordeaux in France. It contains a unique type of bioflavonoid called proanthocyanidins which are synergistic with vitamin C—that is, they greatly enhance the activity of

111

vitamin C. In fact, some researchers believe that pygnogenol helps vitamin C enter cells, thus strengthening the cell membrane and protecting the cells from oxidative damage.

Proanthocyanidins are found in cranberries, grapes, cola nuts and other fruits and vegetables.

THE RIGHT AMOUNT   Pycnogenol is sold in capsule form at health food shops. Take one capsule (30 mg) daily.

POSSIBLE BENEFITS

Cancer Fighter. Pycnogenol is a potent antioxidant and free radical scavenger. Free radicals are unstable oxygen molecules which can attack normal cells, destroying them or causing them to mutate. Free radical damage can also lead to the kind of unfettered cell growth associated with cancer. Vitamin C is a potent antioxidant in its own right, but studies suggest that it may be even more effective when combined with pycnogenol. In fact, according to researchers at the Department of Pharmacy of Nagasaki University School of Medicine, test tube studies showed that the bioflavonoids used in pycnogenol had stronger antioxidant activity than vitamin C.

Heart Disease. Several studies have confirmed that antioxidants like pycnogenol can prevent the oxidation of blood lipids, such as LDL or 'bad' cholesterol, which can promote the formation of plaque or fatty deposits in the arteries.

Anti-inflammatory. Pycnogenol has been used as an anti-inflammatory to treat common ailments such as arthritis and allergies. Many bioflavonoids inhibit the release of certain enzymes that can promote inflammation. In the case of arthritis, free radical damage may also contribute to joint pain and swelling associated with this condition.

Circulation. Capillaries are tiny blood vessels that can be easily destroyed by free radical damage. Also, as we age, cells lose collagen, a protein fibre that is important for the growth and repair of cells, including capillary cells. Weakened capillaries can lead to easy bruising and a tendency to develop varicose veins. Pycnogenol helps strengthen capillaries in two ways. First, by protecting against free radical assault, it may help prevent weakening of capillaries. Secondly, since vitamin C is essential for the production of collagen, and since pycnogenol enhances the performance of vitamin C, it is indirectly involved in collagen production.

QUERCETIN

FACTS Quercetin is a bioflavonoid, a group of compounds found in fruits and vegetables. Many bioflavonoids are now being studied for their ability to prevent disease.

Quercetin, an antioxidant, may also have antiviral properties when combined with vitamin C. Several studies suggest that it may be a potent cancer fighter.

The best food sources of quercetin are yellow and red onions and shallots. High levels are also found in broccoli and Italian squash.

THE RIGHT AMOUNT There is no RDA for quercetin. It is available in supplement form, often in combination with other bioflavonoids or antioxidants. The usual dose is 250 mg, one to two times daily.

POSSIBLE BENEFITS

Cancer Fighter. In many studies, quercetin has been shown to block the action of a variety of natural and synthetic initiators or promoters of cancer cell development. It also appears to inhibit the growth of human tumour cells containing binding sites for type-II oestrogen which may be responsible for some forms of cancer, including breast cancer.

Population studies have shown that people who eat a diet rich in onions and other allium vegetables have substantially lower rates of gastrointestinal cancers than people who don't. Scientists are not precisely sure why onions protect against cancer although they do contain many potentially beneficial phytochemicals, but high levels of quercetin may be a major factor.

Anti-allergy. An allergy is an inflammatory condition triggered by an allergen—any substance, either natural or synthetic, that causes an allergic antibody reaction in the body. In such a reaction, the immune system mistakenly identifies a harmless substance as a dangerous invader and begins to produce chemicals against it, including histamine. Histamine is responsible for sneezing, itchy nose, watery eyes and some of the other unpleasant allergic symptoms. Studies show that quercetin prevents the release of histamine, thus inhibiting the allergic response. Interestingly enough, several other bioflavonoid-like substances are marketed as allergy medications. Quercetin may also be useful against asthma.

REISHI MUSHROOM

FACTS   Ageing takes its toll on the immune system. As people age, their immune systems become less effective at identifying foreign agents and fighting against viruses and bacteria, and as a result, they are more vulnerable to cancer, infections and other related problems. Reishi mushroom, known for its powerful immune-stimulating properties, is one of the most revered herbs in Japan.

THE RIGHT AMOUNT   Reishi is available in capsules at health food shops. Take one capsule up to three times daily. Dried reishi mushrooms can also be bought for use in cooking.

POSSIBLE BENEFITS

Immune Booster. Studies show that compounds found in reishi mushrooms can increase the activity of two types of immune cells which are necessary to fight against potentially troublesome organisms.

Cancer Fighter. Compounds found in reishi mushrooms inhibited the growth of tumours in laboratory mice, which suggests that they may play a similar role in humans.

Heart Disease. Studies show that reishi mushrooms can lower cholesterol and reduce blood pressure.

RESVERATROL

FACTS For centuries people have been drinking each other's good health in an alcoholic beverage and, since biblical times, alcohol, especially wine, has been used as a traditional medicine for a wide range of ailments. In recent years scientists have noticed that moderate drinkers tend to live longer than teetotallers—indeed, in countries like France and Italy, where a glass or two of wine is a routine part of a meal, the incidence of heart disease is much lower than in countries where it is not consumed in such great quantities. Puzzled as to why wine drinkers fared so much better than non-wine drinkers, scientists began to examine the chemistry of wine to see what, if anything, could be providing its beneficial effects. Japanese researchers recently identified an antifungal compound in grape skins, called resveratrol, which lowers the fat content in the livers of rats, thus lowering overall cholesterol. Many scientists believe that resveratrol may have the same effect on humans, which is why a glass or two of wine a day may keep the cardiologist away.

THE RIGHT AMOUNT Drink one or two glasses of wine several times a week. If you are taking any medication, consult your doctor before drinking any alcoholic beverage.

CAUTION Too much wine counteracts any of its potential benefits. People who drink more than one or two glasses of wine per day are putting themselves at risk of developing cardiovascular and liver disease as well as other health problems. If you have a drinking problem, no amount of wine is safe for you.

POSSIBLE BENEFITS

Heart Healthy. Several major studies have confirmed that alcohol in general, and wine in particular, appears to protect against heart disease. A glass or two of wine can lower your blood pressure. Researchers recently discovered that resveratrol and other chemicals in wine are vasodilators—that is, they relax the blood vessels, allowing the blood to flow more easily.

Starting in 1978, a group of researchers at Kaiser Permanente Medical Center in Oakland, California, began a study to determine the effect of alcohol on coronary artery disease. The team collected information on 81,825 men and women. Over the next ten years, the researchers monitored this group for deaths due to heart disease. The results: those who regularly drank alcoholic beverages had a lower rate of death from coronary artery disease, but those who drank wine had the lowest rate of all.

In other studies sponsored by the American Heart Association, people who consumed alcoholic beverages, especially wine, had up to 49 per cent reduction in heart disease compared with those who abstained.

Not only does alcohol appear to cut total cholesterol, but it also raises the rate of beneficial HDLs or 'good' cholesterol. People who drink at least one glass of wine daily have been found to have higher levels of HDL or 'good' cholesterol than non-wine drinkers. This is true for both men and women. In fact, for women, just one glass of wine daily is all it takes to raise HDLs; men require two glasses.

RIBOFLAVIN (VITAMIN B₂)

FACTS   The primary function of this B vitamin is to work with other substances to metabolise carbohydrates, fats and proteins for energy.

Riboflavin may also protect against certain forms of cancer and oxidative damage by free radicals.

People over 55 are at risk of developing a riboflavin deficiency, especially if they do not eat a well-rounded diet and do not take a vitamin supplement.

Good sources of riboflavin include fat-free or low fat dairy products, eggs and leafy vegetables. (Liver is also an excellent source of riboflavin; however, I do not recommend eating liver due to its high cholesterol, high fat content. Toxins—natural and synthetic—are also concentrated in liver.)

THE RIGHT AMOUNT   The RDA for riboflavin is 1.3 to 1.8 mg for adults. Riboflavin is included in most multivitamin supplements, as well as in B-complex supplements. The usual dose is 1–4 mg.

Women who take oestrogen need to take a B_2 supplement.

Riboflavin works best with vitamins B_6, C and niacin.

POSSIBLE BENEFITS

Antioxidant. Riboflavin has antioxidant properties. It also works with the enzyme glutathione reductase to maintain glutathione, which fights against free radical damage. A particularly important role of riboflavin is to protect against oxidative damage during exercise, when the demand for oxygen by the body increases.

Cancer Fighter. Deficiencies of this B vitamin may increase the risk of developing cancer of the oesophagus, especially among people who chew tobacco or drink alcoholic beverages.

Healthy Eyes. Riboflavin can help prevent damage to the cornea of the eye, which can result in cataracts.

Boosts Immunity. Riboflavin deficiency can decrease the number of T-cells, an important component of the immune system. Low levels of T-cells may increase the risk of developing cancer and other diseases.

For Active Women. Studies show that active older women may require higher levels of riboflavin than the RDA. Researchers at Cornell University recently studied the effect of riboflavin levels on exercise in women aged 60–67. For eight weeks, these women exercised for up to 25 minutes daily on a stationary bicycle. Half the group was given the RDA for riboflavin, the other half was given 150 per cent of the RDA. Blood levels of B_2 dropped in the women who were given only the RDA. Researchers concluded that older women who exercise regularly may need extra riboflavin.

SAW PALMETTO

FACTS   The Native Americans ate the berries of the saw palmetto plant by the handful. Known by the botanical name *Serenoa repens*, naturopaths and herbalists in the United States and Europe have long used saw palmetto berries to treat problems of the genito-urinary tract in both sexes. In fact, saw palmetto is a folk remedy for so-called 'honeymoon cystitis', a condition caused by too much sexual activity. This herb was also touted as an aphrodisiac. Today, in Germany, extract of saw palmetto is a leading treatment for benign prostate hypertrophy (enlarged prostate), and is reputed to be so successful that American doctors are taking a second look at this 'archaic' medicine.

THE RIGHT AMOUNT Saw palmetto is available in extract or capsule form at most health food shops and herbalists. Mix 30–60 drops in liquid daily, or take one to three capsules.

POSSIBLE BENEFITS

Prostate. In men, the prostate gland is a walnut-size organ surrounding the urethra, which is located at the neck of the bladder. By the age of 50, most men develop a slightly enlarged prostate, a benign condition which can result in excessive urination, especially at night, or difficulty in passing urine. Benign prostate hypertrophy is believed to be caused by an excess build-up of testosterone, the male hormone, in the prostate. This excess is converted into dihydrotestosterone, a more potent form of the hormone that can promote cell growth, thus leading to the enlargement. Excess levels of testosterone are also believed to be linked to cancer of the prostate. Several scientific studies have shown that saw palmetto extracts can alter the biological pathways that lead to the conversion of testosterone to its more potent form, dihydrotestosterone. In addition, by preventing the more potent testosterone from binding to receptor sites on the cells, it may help rid the body of this potentially dangerous hormone.

Saw palmetto may not only help to prevent enlargement of the prostate, but has proved to be an effective treatment for this condition. In a 1984 study published in the *British Journal of Pharmacology*, 110 patients suffering from enlarged prostate were given either saw palmetto extract or a placebo for 30 days. Patients on saw palmetto experienced a significant reduction in symptoms, such as fewer night-time urinations (down by 45 per cent) and improved urine flow. Those on the placebo showed little change in their condition.

PERSONAL ADVICE   If you have discomfort or difficulty with urination, or pass blood with your urine, consult your doctor. Do not self-diagnose. However, if your doctor confirms that you have benign prostate hypertrophy, try using saw palmetto to see if it helps. If you don't see any improvement within a month or so, talk to your doctor about medication. New drug treatments have been quite effective in treating enlarged prostate, but saw palmetto extract may work just as well in some cases.

SCHIZANDRA

FACTS   This highly prized Chinese herb is fast becoming a best seller in the United States because of its reputation as a longevity herb and aphrodisiac. Since ancient times schizandra has been favoured among the wealthy Chinese. Until recently it has been rare and expensive, but today it is widely available in China and the United States. Herbal healers have used schizandra to treat lung disorders, and recent studies show that extracts from this herb are effective against the bacteria that cause tuberculosis.

Similar to ginseng, schizandra is believed to increase stamina and relieve fatigue. It is also used to treat stress and depression. According to one study, polo horses given schizandra performed better and showed better physiological responses to stress after taking the herb.

THE RIGHT AMOUNT   Schizandra is available in capsules at some health food shops. Take one to three capsules daily. It can also be obtained from specialists in Chinese medicine.

POSSIBLE BENEFITS

Liver. Animal studies have shown that this herb can help protect the liver from toxins, thus helping to preserve this vital organ.

Aphrodisiac. In China, schizandra is highly regarded as an aphrodisiac for both sexes. According to Ron Teeguarden, author of *Chinese Tonic Herbs*, 'It relieves fatigue and is quite famous for increasing the sexual staying power in men.' Teeguarden notes, schizandra does no less for women, adding, 'it causes the female genitals to feel warm, healthy and extremely sensitive.'

SEAWEED

FACTS   Seaweed is a primitive, plant-like organism that grows in the sea. It is a dietary mainstay in Japan and was traditionally gathered for food around the coasts of the British Isles.

Dietary seaweed is sold in oriental and health food shops. There are several varieties of seaweed or algae, differentiated by their colour. Nori, a red seaweed, is used to wrap sushi. Popular forms of brown seaweed include kelp, wakame, arme and kombu.

Traditional Chinese healers have used hot water extracts of seaweed to treat cancer and recent studies show that compounds in seaweed may indeed protect against cancer.

THE RIGHT AMOUNT   There is no RDA or study that specifies the correct amount of seaweed needed to prevent cancer. However, in Japan, where the cancer rate is a fraction of that in the West, most people eat some form of seaweed daily. In fact, the estimated *per capita* intake of seaweed in Japan ranges from 4.9–7.3 grams daily.

POSSIBLE BENEFITS

Cancer Fighter. Japanese scientists isolated several polysaccharides, potentially anticarcinogenic compounds, in seaweed. One of these, fucoidin, may prove to be a potent cancer fighter. Several studies show that these compounds may have a dramatic impact on cancer. In one study, laboratory mice were injected with cancer cells. One group of mice received an extract from marine algae, the other group was given water without the extract. The life span of the treated mice was 37 per cent longer than that of the control animals. Researchers speculate that the seaweed may somehow boost the body's immunological defences against tumour growth. However, test tube studies also show that seaweed extract can prevent or slow down the growth of cancer cells outside the body, which suggests that it may also inhibit the growth of cells on its own.

SELENIUM

FACTS Not until the 1950s did researchers recognise that this mineral played a vital role in the human body. In recent years, selenium has become a superstar among minerals because of its reputed ability to prevent cancer and heart disease.

Selenium is an antioxidant. It works with glutathione peroxidase to prevent damage by free radicals. Selenium is also involved in the metabolism of prostaglandins, hormonelike substances used by the body in many different ways.

In the body, selenium detoxifies metal such as arsenic and mercury, which would otherwise be lethal.

Selenium is synergistic with vitamin E, which means that the two combined increase the potency of each other.

Good food sources of selenium include garlic, onions, tuna, herring, broccoli, wheat germ, whole grains, sesame seeds, red grapes, egg yolks and mushrooms. The selenium content in food varies from region to region due to differing levels of selenium in the soil.

THE RIGHT AMOUNT The RDA is 150–200 mcg daily. I recommend 200 mcg daily, but some cancer researchers feel that 300 mcg per day are needed. Selenium can be toxic in high doses, so do not exceed 300 mcg daily. (Studies have shown that toxicity may occur at levels of 2400 mcg daily for a prolonged period of time. However, I suggest that we err on the side of caution until we know precisely what levels are safe.

POSSIBLE BENEFITS

Cancer Fighter. Population studies show that the death rate from cancer can be directly correlated to the selenium intake of food—people who eat the least amount of selenium have the highest rates of cancer. For example, in Japan, where the daily selenium intake is 500 mcg, the cancer rate is more than five times lower than it is in countries where the selenium intake is half that amount. Researchers have also found higher blood levels of selenium in healthy people than in cancer patients.

Many animal studies confirm that selenium can prevent cancerous growths. Some studies show that it actually protects cell membranes from attack by free radicals which may explain its ability to ward off cancer.

Cardiovascular Health. Selenium may protect lipids from oxidation, a process that may contribute to the formation of atherosclerotic lesions in the coronary arteries, and it may also help to prevent blood clots which can cause a stroke. Studies have linked a low selenium intake to a higher rate of both heart attack and stroke. In Colorado Springs, Colorado, which boasts the highest selenium soil content in the United States, the death rate due to heart disease is 67 per cent below the national average.

Anti-inflammatory. Selenium appears to have some anti-inflammatory properties. In combination with vitamin E, it has been used to treat arthritis in animal studies. Some people swear that selenium can help reduce the pain and stiffness of arthritis.

Male Potency. Men need this mineral! Selenium is necessary for sperm production. Almost half of a male's supply of selenium is concentrated in the testicles and portions of the seminal ducts adjacent to the prostate gland. Selenium is reputed to increase the male sex drive.

SESAME

FACTS No reputable Asian chef would be caught without his or her bottle of sesame oil, a commonly used seasoning in oriental cooking. Asians may use sesame oil because of its delicate, nutty flavour, but Westerners could well turn to it as a painless way to help prevent cancer and heart disease.

THE RIGHT AMOUNT Sprinkle a few drops of sesame oil on stir-fry dishes.

POSSIBLE BENEFITS

Anti-cancer. Sesame seeds and oil are an excellent source of phytic acid, an antioxidant that may prevent the kind of cellular damage that can lead to cancer. Japanese studies have shown that sesame oil may protect against colon cancer. In animal studies, sesame oil added to the diet of rats reduced the amount of bile acids in the faeces. Bile acids are believed to produce cancerous changes in cells of the intestinal wall, which could cause colon cancer.

Heart Disease. Sesamin, a lignin from sesame oil, significantly reduced the amount of serum and liver cholesterol in rats fed a normal diet. Researchers speculate that sesamin may help keep cholesterol levels under control in humans.

SOLANACEOUS FOODS

FACTS Mediterranean regions, such as Crete and mainland Greece, have a much lower rate of heart disease and cancer than in the West. Perhaps the people there can attribute their good health to their high intake of solanaceous foods. The solanaceous family, which includes tomatoes, aubergine and peppers, is being investigated by the American National Cancer Institute for its potential cancer-preventive properties. These foods are a mainstay of Mediterranean cuisine, and are found in abundance at nearly every meal. Solanaceous foods are also an excellent source of vitamins, minerals and fibre.

THE RIGHT AMOUNT I recommend eating at least one serving of solanaceous food daily. You cannot get these critical phytochemicals in a vitamin pill, you must eat the whole food!

CAUTION Some people with arthritis may find that peppers and tomatoes may aggravate their condition.

POSSIBLE BENEFITS

Cancer Fighter. Out of the fourteen possible phytochemicals known or believed to possess anti-cancer activity, the solanaceous family has seven of these important compounds including flavonoids, glucarates, carotenoids, coumarins, mono-terpenes, tri-terpenes, and phenolic acids. Researchers believe that each of these compounds may intercede at various stages of cancer development. Some compounds may block a carcinogen that can initiate cancer—that is, a substance which alters a healthy cell, making it susceptible to cancerous growth. Others may block a cancer promoter, the substance which stimulates the altered cell to grow.

SOYA BEANS

FACTS The American National Cancer Institute is giving top priority to investigating the potential cancer-fighting properties of soya beans, and several studies have shown that soya may protect against heart disease. Anyone who wants to live longer should be eating this food.

The Japanese, who live longer than any other nationality on earth, eat lots of soya, and some researchers believe that this longevity may be due to the fact that the typical Japanese diet is rich in soya foods, products derived from soya beans. Tofu, a beancurd made from dried soya beans, and miso, a soup made from soya paste, are staples in the Japanese diet.

Ironically the United States, not Japan, is the world's leading producer of soya. Although it is not as popular in the West as it is in Japan, soya-based foods are to be found in health food shops and supermarkets throughout Britain, Europe and the United States. Rich in protein, soya is an extremely versatile food that can be used in many different ways. Soya 'milk' is used in formula for infants who are allergic to cow's milk. Rehydrated textured vegetable protein, a soya product sold in health food

124

shops, can be used as a substitute for minced beef. Soya flour can be used in baking and as a thickener. Tofu, which is flavourless and odourless, takes on the flavour of other foods and spices and can be made into everything from a frozen dessert resembling ice cream to a mock 'egg' salad.

THE RIGHT AMOUNT   I recommend eating at least one soya product daily.

POSSIBLE BENEFITS

Heart Disease. Recent studies show that adding soya to your diet may be one of the most effective ways of lowering cholesterol. A group headed by researcher Susan M. Potter, at the University of Illinois in Urbana-Champaign, tested the effects of soya protein consumption on 26 men with moderately high cholesterol. The men replaced 50 per cent of their normal daily protein consumption with 50 grams of soya protein. The protein was baked into foods such as muffins, biscuits and breads. At the end of four weeks, each man had an average reduction in total cholesterol of 12 per cent, thus reducing their risk of heart disease by 25 per cent.

Although soya is not typically used as a cholesterol-lowering treatment, according to Dr Potter it is the primary cholesterol reduction treatment in Italy. Based on the study at the University of Illinois, it appears that soya protein may be as effective a treatment as some of the medications that are prescribed for hypercholesterolaemia, which have many dangerous and unpleasant side effects. If you have high cholesterol, you may want to talk to your doctor about trying a soya regime before taking medication.

Cancer Fighter. There are several compounds in soya that may help to prevent cancer. Soya contains phytochemicals called lignans and isoflavonoids, two compounds that are converted in the intestine into an oestrogen-like substance called *ekuol*. This competes with a more potent form of oestrogen, oestradiol, for space on oestrogen receptors on some cells. If the oestradiol has nowhere to bind, it becomes deactivated. Many researchers believe that oestradiol promotes the growth of tumours, especially in the breast. Significantly, Japanese women, who typically eat lots of soya, have a much lower rate of breast cancer than women in the West.

Soya may have a similar effect on the hormonal balance in men. Prostate cancer, far more common in the West than in Japan, is believed to be caused by high levels of a potent form of testosterone, which may be deactivated by lignans and iso-flavonoids. There may be other factors contributing to the disparity in cancer—Japanese men eat a diet that is much lower in fat and red meat—but the phytochemicals in soya may also offer some protection.

Genistein is another compound in soya that is believed to be a potent cancer fighter. Genistein blocks angiogenesis, the process in which new blood vessels grow, thus literally 'starving' malignant tumours from the nutrients needed to help them grow.

Menopause Aid. In Japan, hot flushes and other unpleasant symptoms of menopause due to lower oestrogen levels are a rarity, and few Japanese women take Hormone Replacement Therapy, a common treatment for menopause in the West. Soya researcher Herman Aldercreutz, of the University of Helsinki, suggested in a letter to the *New England Journal of Medicine* that the hormone-like properties of the phytochemicals in soya may be one reason why Japanese women have an easier time with menopause than women in the West.

SULPHORAPHANE

FACTS Sulphoraphane is a phytochemical, a biologically active compound found in many cruciferous vegetables (broccoli, brussels sprouts, kale, cauliflower) and also in carrots and green onions. According to researchers at Johns Hopkins School of Medicine, sulphoraphane may be the most powerful natural anti-cancer compound discovered to date.

THE RIGHT AMOUNT There is no RDA for sulphoraphane. I recommend two servings of sulphoraphane-rich foods daily.

POSSIBLE BENEFITS

Anti-cancer. Vegetables contain chemicals that promote the formation of different enzymes in humans. Some of these enzymes (Phase 1) are 'villains'—they actually convert benign substances into oxidants, which can damage a cell's DNA, thus promoting the risk of cancer. In response to the oxidant threat, cells can also make Phase II enzymes, the so-called 'heroes' who protect the cells' vulnerable genetic material from the 'villains'. Many foods, such as hamburgers, cause cells to create both good and bad enzymes. However, researchers at Johns Hopkins discovered that sulphoraphane promotes the production of only Phase II 'good' enzymes, thus helping the body to ward off potential carcinogens. Although there may be other foods that also trigger the production of only Phase II enzymes, the researchers suspect that sulphoraphane may create even higher levels of good enzymes than these other foods.

In animal studies, sulphoraphane has been shown to protect against cancer. In one study, scientists pretreated 29 rats with a synthetic version of sulphoraphane and then injected them with a carcinogen known to induce mammary tumours. The scientists then injected 25 other rats with the carcinogen without pretreating them with the sulphoraphane. More than two-thirds of the group that did not receive the sulphoraphane treatment eventually developed mammary cancers compared with only 35 per cent of the group that received a low dose of sulphoraphane. Of the rats that received a high dose of sulphoraphane, only 26 per cent went on to develop cancer.

More studies are needed to determine if sulphoraphane will have the same effect on women.

THIAMIN (VITAMIN B₁)

FACTS   Thiamin, known as Vitamin B_1, breaks down and converts carbohydrates into glucose, which provides energy for the body. Thiamin is necessary for the normal functioning of the nervous system, heart and other muscles.

Gross thiamin deficiency will lead to beriberi, a life-threatening disease that used commonly to afflict sailors. Today beriberi is rare, but mild thiamin deficiency is common among older people and can lead to lack of energy, moodiness, numbness in the legs, mild depression, loss of appetite and a general apathy, among other symptoms.

Good food sources of thiamin include brewer's yeast, rice husks, unrefined cereal grains, sunflower seeds, pecans, lean pork, green peas, offal, most vegetables and milk. However, it is easily destroyed by exposure to light and heat

THE RIGHT AMOUNT The RDA for thiamin for adults is 1.0 to 1.5 mg. Thiamin can be destroyed by alcohol, and therefore alcoholics and heavy drinkers are at risk of thiamin deficiency. Thiamin is usually included in B-complex supplements and multivitamins.

If you use antacids or aspirin on a regular basis, you may need extra thiamin.

Thiamin has no known toxic effects.

POSSIBLE BENEFITS

Heart Disease. Thiamin is essential for the normal function of the heart and serious deficiencies may lead to potentially fatal heart arrhythmias and heart failure. Given the fact that heart disease is the number one killer in America and Britain, and that studies show thiamin deficiency to be not uncommon among the elderly, it is critical for older adults to maintain normal thiamin levels.

Anti-stress. In times of physical or emotional stress your intake of B vitamins, including thiamin, should be increased. In my experience, many people find that thiamin along with other B vitamins, can help alleviate symptoms of stress such as mild depression.

TOCOPHEROL (VITAMIN E)

FACTS A doctor friend, who is highly sceptical about all forms of vitamin supplements, recently confessed that she is beginning to have second thoughts about vitamin E. 'I've noticed that

128

among my older patients, those who take vitamin E are the most together, healthiest people in my practice,' she said. 'It finally dawned on me that there must be something to this vitamin E.'

A lot of people, many of them medical practitioners, have reached the same conclusion. Sales of vitamin E have soared, and it is now enjoying superstar status among its fellow micronutrients. However, vitamin E is no overnight success: it took more than 70 years for the medical community to begin to take it seriously.

Vitamin E was first discovered in 1922, when researchers noticed, quite by accident, that rats could not breed without it. They dubbed this substance tocopherol, from the Greek 'to bring forth in childbirth'. There are actually eight different types of tocopherol, of which alpha tocopherol is the most effective.

Vitamin E is a fat soluble vitamin, which means that, unlike water soluble vitamins, it is not excreted in the urine but is stored in the liver.

Vitamin E is a potent antioxidant; it has been dubbed the body's first line of defence against lipid peroxidation—that means it protects polyunsaturated fatty acids in the cell membrane from free radical attack.

Vitamin E is found in vegetable oils, whole grains, sweet potato, wheat germ, brown rice, nuts and other foods.

It is synergistic with selenium (another 'Hot Hundred' antioxidant) which means that the two combined greatly enhance each other's potency.

THE RIGHT AMOUNT The RDA for vitamin E is 10 mg or 14.9 iu, but supplements usually come in 200 or 400 iu strength. I recommend at least 400 iu of vitamin E daily.

CAUTION Do not take vitamin E if you are taking a blood thinner such as aspirin, or have vitamin K deficiency. If you have had a bleeding problem in the past, talk to your doctor before taking vitamin E.

POSSIBLE BENEFITS

Heart Disease. In the 1970s two Canadian doctors, Drs Wilfred and Evan Shute, promoted vitamin E as a weapon against heart disease in their best-selling book, *Vitamin E for Ailing and Healthy Hearts.* Most cardiologists ridiculed the notion that a mere vitamin could be powerful heart medicine. They are no longer laughing. Several recent studies have shown a link between daily vitamin E consumption and a lowered risk of heart disease in both men and women. In May 1993 the *New England Journal of Medicine* reported the results of an eight-year study involving more than 87,000 registered female nurses and a related study involving close to 40,000 male health professionals. In both studies, participants who consumed vitamin E supplements (of at least 100 iu or more) for a minimum of two years had a 40 per cent lower risk of heart disease than those who derived vitamin E through diet alone. At first, researchers suspected that people taking vitamin E might be more health-conscious and therefore have healthier habits, which could also account for the reduction in heart disease. However, even after making allowances for lifestyle, the vitamin E supplement appeared to be the primary difference between the group who got heart disease and the group who remained disease free.

In another study, sponsored by the American Heart Association, researchers found that long-term supplementation with high doses of vitamin E (160mg) decreased LDL or 'bad' cholesterol susceptibility to oxidation by 30 to 50 per cent. When LDL becomes oxidised, it may contribute to the formation of atherosclerotic lesions in arteries supplying blood to the heart and other vital organs. A heart attack occurs when blood supply is cut off from the heart.

Vitamin E is also a natural blood thinner, and may prevent the formation of blood clots. If a clot enters the bloodstream and lodges in an artery feeding the brain, it could result in a stroke; if the clot lodges into a coronary artery, it could result in a heart attack.

Many cardiac surgeons give coronary by-pass patients high doses of vitamin E prior to surgery. A recent study of coronary by-pass patients performed at the Mayo Clinic in Rochester,

Minnesota, found that patients given 2000 iu vitamin E prior to surgery had much lower blood levels of free radicals after surgery than patients who had not been given the supplement. They also found that patients who had been given additional vitamin E had normal blood levels of E following surgery, while the unsupplemented patients had lower than normal levels.

Cancer Fighter. There is growing evidence that vitamin E may protect against various forms of cancer. A study sponsored by the American National Cancer Institute suggests that people who take a vitamin E supplement for a minimum of six months cut their risk of developing oral cancers by half. Factors known to increase the risk of oral cancers, such as alcohol consumption, smoking and dietary habits—made no difference in the outcome. These findings are consistent with animal studies that showed that vitamin E reduced the effects of carcinogens on cheek cells in hamsters.

Another study performed at the Biodynamics Institute at Louisiana State University showed that vitamin E may protect humans against the harmful effects of chronic exposure to ozone in smog. The study suggests that vitamin E's potent antioxidant activity may guard against the biological damage inflicted by ozone on lung tissue.

Vitamin E may also help to prevent stomach cancer and other cancers of the gastrointestinal tract by inhibiting the conversion of nitrates, which are found in food, to nitrosamines in the stomach. Nitrosamines are potentially carcinogenic.

Diabetes. In a recent Italian study, daily vitamin E supplements (900 mg for four months) helped people with Type II diabetes use insulin better. Type II diabetes—also known as adult or late onset diabetes—accounts for 90 per cent of all cases of diabetes and occurs during middle age and beyond. People with this form of diabetes can develop dangerously high levels of glucose in the blood. Based on this study, vitamin E appeared to help maintain normal blood glucose levels. (If you have diabetes, consult your doctor before using vitamin E or any other medication.)

Immunity. Studies have shown that older people with low

131

blood serum levels of vitamin E are more vulnerable to developing infections. A recent study in the *American Journal of Clinical Nutrition* showed that short-term supplementation with high doses of vitamin E can enhance immune responsiveness in healthy individuals over the age of 60. In the study, 32 healthy older adults who were not taking any vitamin supplements or prescription medication were either given 800 mg of vitamin E daily for three days, or a placebo. Based on blood and skin tests, those taking the vitamin E showed a dramatic boost in immune function. Those taking the placebo did not show any change. Considering the fact that immune function declines as we age, this is a particularly important finding.

Brain. Researchers at the Neurological Institute at Columbia University College of Physicians and Surgeons in New York gave patients with tardive dyskinesia (a neurological disorder that can result from long-term use of anti-psychotic medications) vitamin E supplements as well as their anti-psychotic medications. The group taking the vitamin E showed improvement in tremors and a reduction in anxiety and depression. Researchers are considering using antioxidant vitamins, including E, on patients with Parkinson's disease, another neurologic disorder that often affects the elderly.

Skin. For decades vitamin E fans have claimed that, if used directly on the skin, vitamin E oil can help prevent the signs of ageing. A recent study suggests that vitamin E may indeed reduce the severity of wrinkles. In the study, 20 middle-aged women were given a five per cent strength cream of vitamin E to put on their skin daily. At the end of four weeks, the women showed a 50 per cent reduction in the length and depth of crow's feet— although the wrinkles were still there, they looked better. However, many cosmetic creams that tout vitamin E as an ingredient actually contain very little. Use only creams that list vitamin E or tocopherol near the top of the ingredients label, which means that it is a primary ingredient. Do not use the oil from a vitamin E capsule directly on the skin—it can cause irritation in many people.

Protects Against Muscle Damage. Although vigorous exercise

132

is good for your heart, it may also promote muscle damage due to oxidation. (Remember that, as you exercise, your body's demand for oxygen increases—the more oxygen, the greater the risk of oxidation.) However, according to a study at the Human Nutrition Research Center on Aging at Tufts University, a daily vitamin E supplement may help protect against free radical damage caused by working out.

Eyes. Researchers suspect that cataracts, which cloud the eye lens, may be caused by oxidative damage to the lens covering of the eye, and that vitamin E may help protect the eye from this kind of damage. A recent study suggests that they may be right. Finnish researchers discovered that people with low blood serum levels of vitamin E (and also beta-carotene, another member of the Hot Hundred) were twice as likely to develop cataracts as those with higher levels.

Arthritis. Studies suggest that vitamin E supplements may relieve some of the symptoms of osteoarthritis. Arthritis has been associated with elevated levels of free radicals.

Anecdotal Evidence. Many people swear that vitamin E helps to prevent their hair from turning grey. Recently, an Ohio doctor even wrote a letter to the *New York Times* describing how he and his patients keep their hair from turning grey by taking vitamin E. Although there is no evidence to prove that vitamin E helps to keep the grey away, I have heard it from enough people to make me wonder whether there is any truth in it.

TRETINOIN

FACTS Marketed under the name Retin-A, tretinoin, a form of topical vitamin A, is an approved treatment for severe acne. Dermatologists have observed that this cream not only helps rid their patients of acne, but appears to help erase fine lines and wrinkles. In the late 1980s tretinoin was being touted as a miracle cream and quickly became one of the most frequently prescribed topical medications. In recent years it has been eclipsed by the growing popularity of alpha-hydroxy acids and other hot, new 'cosmeceuticals'. Tretinoin has its shortcomings: its effectiveness peaks after about 24 months of use. In addition, if you stop using it, the changes begin to fade. Despite these problems, tretinoin is still one of the most effective anti-ageing skin products on the market.

THE RIGHT AMOUNT Apply cream as directed by your doctor.

CAUTION Most users experience skin peeling or irritation at least initially. Tretinoin must be used in conjunction with a sunscreen because it makes the skin more prone to sun damage. High doses of oral vitamin A have been associated with birth defects. Although there is no evidence that topical vitamin A can cause similar problems, women who are pregnant or trying to conceive should not use tretinoin.

POSSIBLE BENEFITS

Skin Rejuvenator. As we age, skin tends to thin out and become drier. Wrinkles develop when collagen and elastin, proteins in the skin that provide elasticity, begin to break down. Studies have shown that tretinoin can increase skin thickness, improve circulation and increase collagen. (Collagen is the 'glue' that holds cells together.) Tretinoin appears to help plump out the skin, erasing fine lines and wrinkles. After about six weeks of use, many people find that their skins look pinker and fresher. (However, tretinoin is ineffective against deep wrinkles.)

TURMERIC

FACTS Turmeric is a herb that adds flavour and colour to many foods, including curry powder and sauces. In the West it has been used primarily as a spice, but in Asia this herb has a rich medicinal history. Westerners are just beginning to discover its potential as a longevity booster.

Turmeric is a 'heart-healthy' herb that may help prevent heart disease. It is also a natural anti-inflammatory.

THE RIGHT AMOUNT   Turmeric is available in capsule and tablet form. Take one to three capsules or tablets daily.

POSSIBLE BENEFITS

Heart Disease. Studies show that turmeric can lower blood cholesterol levels. It stimulates the production of bile by the liver and, since cholesterol is a component of bile, when the liver produces bile it utilises excess cholesterol.

Turmeric also prevents the formation of dangerous blood clots that can lead to heart attack or stroke. As Daniel Mowrey noted in his book, *Next Generation Herbal Medicine*, people who live in countries where curry is frequently eaten have a much lower incidence of thrombosis (blood clots) than people who live in Western countries.

Arthritis. Traditional healers have used turmeric to reduce the inflammation and pain associated with arthritis. Based on anecdotal evidence, I believe that some people may find that turmeric may indeed help control arthritis.

UNBELLIFEROUS VEGETABLES

FACTS   In an article that appeared in *Food Technology*, Dr Alegria Caragay, an adviser to the 'Designer Food Programme' for the American National Cancer Institute, wrote, 'Within the last decade, as research into the relationship between diet and cancer has proliferated, so, too, has the body of data from both epidemiological and animal studies that indicates vegetables, grains, and fruits may contain certain cancer-preventing substances.' In the article, Dr Caragay noted that umbelliferous vegetables were at the top of the NCI's list of foods with potentially important anti-cancer properties—indeed, the NCI is pouring millions of dollars into researching these foods.

Unbelliferous vegetables include carrots, celery and parsnips.

THE RIGHT AMOUNT   Unbelliferous vegetables contain six important phytochemicals that may help prevent cancer and heart disease. You cannot get these compounds in a pill, you must eat the whole food. People who want to live longer and stay healthier should make sure that unbelliferous vegetables are included in their diets.

POSSIBLE BENEFITS

Cancer Fighter. Unbelliferous vegetables contain compounds that can thwart the initiation and spread of cancer. They include:

- Flavonoids. These compounds help protect cell membranes against oxidation and may deactivate potent hormones that can trigger the growth of tumours.
- Carotenoids. These compounds help protect cells against oxidative damage that can harm DNA.
- Coumarins. These compounds may block the action of carcinogens before they can damage healthy cells, which can cause these cells to mutate.
- Phenolic acids. These compounds may block the action of hormonelike compounds called prostaglandins which can promote the growth of tumours.

Heart Disease. Umbelliferous vegetables are rich in antioxidants such as carotenoids (beta-carotene), flavonoids and phenolic acids. Studies have shown that people who take antioxidants daily have lower rates of heart disease than those who do not, and researchers believe that antioxidants may prevent the oxidation of LDL or 'bad' cholesterol which may promote atherosclerosis or 'hardening of the arteries'.

VITAMIN D (CALCIFEROL)

FACTS Calcitrol (also called vitamin D) is known as the sunshine vitamin because the ultraviolet B rays of the sun trigger oils of the skin to produce this vitamin. Calcitrol can also be obtained through food. Vitamin D works with calcium and phosphorus to produce strong bones.

The risk of vitamin D deficiency increases with age. Many sunscreens screen out the rays that produce vitamin D and also, as we age, our bodies are less able to convert vitamin D into the active hormone that is needed for dietary calcium to become incorporated into bones. If you do not eat a diet rich in vitamin D, and if you avoid exposure to the sun (which is wise considering the high rate of skin cancer), you may not be getting enough of this vitamin.

Good food sources of vitamin D are fortified low fat or fat free dairy products, and fatty fish such as sardines, mackerel, salmon and tuna.

THE RIGHT AMOUNT The RDA for adults is 5 mcg or 200 iu, but a recent study suggested that women need 500 iu of vitamin D during the winter to prevent bone loss. Talk to your doctor or natural healer about taking a vitamin D supplement.

CAUTION Excessively high doses of vitamin D can be toxic.

POSSIBLE BENEFITS

Osteoporosis. Decreased activity and less exposure to sun can result in wintertime bone loss, but according to one study conducted by Tufts University, a vitamin D supplement may help to prevent this loss. In the study, 249 healthy postmenopausal women with a dietary intake of about 100 iu of vitamin D daily were selected to receive a calcium supplement of 800 mg/dl daily. One half of the group were given an additional supplement of 400 iu of vitamin D daily. The rest were given a placebo. Researchers then measured the patients' spinal bone mineral density in the summer months and in the winter months. As expected, women in both groups showed an increase in spinal bone mineral density in the summer, but the women taking the vitamin D supplement showed significantly less bone loss during the winter than those taking the placebo. Based on this study, it would seem wise to take at least 400 iu of vitamin D daily in addition to eating a calcium rich diet.

VITEX

FACTS Vitex, a herb that dates back to ancient times, is being rediscovered by a generation of modern women who are seeking a natural approach to menopause. Also called the chaste tree or chasteberry, or by its Latin name, *Vitex agnus-castus*, vitex was used by the early Greeks who believed that it could dampen sexual desire. According to *The New Age Herbalist*, in Italy the flowers of this plant are still strewn in the path of novices when they first enter the monastery or convent, presumably because of vitex's reputation as an anti-aphrodisiac. Folklore aside, although there is no evidence that vitex has any effect whatsoever on libido, this herb does appear to have a positive effect on the female reproductive system and is used to treat a wide variety of 'female complaints'.

THE RIGHT AMOUNT Vitex is available in capsule or tablet form at health food shops (you may find it sold as Agnus Castus). Take one capsule or tablet up to three times daily. Vitex is also included in many herbal formulae for women.

POSSIBLE BENEFITS

Menopause. Herbalists have traditionally used vitex to treat symptoms associated with menstrual problems such as PMS. Recent studies show that vitex is a 'hormone regulator'. It increases production of luteinising hormone, inhibits production of follicle-stimulating hormone and may stimulate the production of progesterone. The overall effect of vitex is to prevent the kind of hormonal fluctuations that can cause some very annoying symptoms during menopause, such as hot flushes and irritability.

WATER

FACTS Most of us take water for granted, yet we couldn't live without it for more than a few days. Water is involved in nearly every bodily process and is the most abundant mineral in the human body, accounting for one-half to two-thirds of total body weight.

Nutrients and hormones circulate throughout the body via water. Water also improves kidney function, which tends to decline with age. In addition, water cushions or lubricates joints and prevents friction between bones and ligaments.

Water is also an excellent source of minerals such as calcium, magnesium and selenium. The rate of cardiovascular disease is higher in areas with 'soft water', that is, where the water contains low levels of minerals such as magnesium and calcium.

As we age, our sensation of thirst becomes somewhat blunted, which increases the risk of not drinking enough fluids.

Good sources of water include drinking water, juices, milk, fruits and vegetables. Watermelon, lettuce, cucumber and celery are especially good sources.

THE RIGHT AMOUNT   I advise six to eight glasses of water daily. Be sure to drink water even if you're not thirsty.

CAUTION   Unfortunately, not all water is pure and healthy. In some cases it may be tainted with lead from old pipes; in others, high levels of chlorine and other potential toxins may make it unsafe. If you live in an area where the water is suspect, I recommend installing a home filtering system or using bottled water for drinking.

If you use a home filtering system, remember that it must be properly maintained and checked periodically. Activated carbon filters must be changed every few months or they can develop harmful contaminants. If you have a reverse osmosis system (which removes chemicals but not necessarily all inorganic contaminants), be sure to test it periodically because the filter can become tainted with bacteria. Distillers, which are excellent for removing inorganic contaminants (but not quite as good for organic contaminants) must be descaled regularly.

Depending on processing techniques, not all bottled water is safe either. To ensure purity, try to use only water that has undergone the process of reverse osmosis, distillation or a combination of reverse osmosis and deionisation. Stick to well-known or national brands.

POSSIBLE BENEFITS

Prevents Constipation. Older people spend a lot of money every year on laxatives. Drinking six to eight glasses of water per day will help to increase intestinal motility and prevent constipation.

Weight Control. Instead of reaching for something to eat, try drinking a glass of water. If you're dieting, drink a glass or two of water before meals to curb your appetite. Water fills you up without filling you out.

Skin. As we age, sweat and oil glands, which moisturise skin, begin to slow down. The top layer of skin begins to thin, which makes it more difficult for skin to retain its natural moisture, resulting in drier, older-looking skin, and if you don't replace fluid lost to urination and sweat, your body will pull fluid from other body cells, including skin cells. Drinking water can help your skin retain some of its youthful freshness.

PERSONAL ADVICE If you're running a fever, you need to be sure to drink enough water. Also, if you drink a lot of coffee, tea or colas with caffeine, be sure to increase your water intake since caffeine is a natural diuretic that can increase water loss.

WHEAT BRAN

FACTS All bran is not the same. Researchers are discovering that different kinds of bran perform different functions in the body. Some types are particularly good at lowering cholesterol, others promote bowel regularity. Because of its unique properties, wheat bran may protect against two common forms of cancer, breast cancer and colon cancer.

Good sources of wheat bran include whole wheat bread and cereals. Wheat bran can also be added to hot cereal or baked foods, or mixed in yogurt.

THE RIGHT AMOUNT I recommend one to two servings of a food rich in wheat bran daily.

POSSIBLE BENEFITS

Breast Cancer. Higher levels of circulating oestrogen are believed to be a risk factor for developing breast cancer. Recently, researchers at the American Health Foundation studied the effect of three different types of bran (oat, maize and wheat) on the oestrogen levels of sixty-two premenopausal women. Participants were randomly selected to receive either a wheat, oat or maize bran supplement in the form of food. For each woman, the average daily fibre intake was increased from about 15 to 30 per cent. After two months, the women taking the maize or oat bran showed no change in oestrogen levels. The women eating the diet rich in wheat bran, however, showed significant reductions in serone oestrone, a potent form of oestrogen that may promote the growth of oestrogen-sensitive tumours.

Colon Cancer. Although some forms of colon cancer may be genetic, most appear to be due to diet and environmental factors. A recent study at New York Hospital/Cornell Medical Center suggests that wheat bran may play an important part in preventing this disease. In the study, 58 people with precancerous polyps were divided into two groups. One group was put on a high fibre diet rich in wheat bran cereal. The other group was given a low fibre cereal. Most of the people eating the wheat bran experienced a reduction in the size and number of their polyps. There was no change seen in those on the low fibre diet.

WHITE WILLOW

FACTS For thousands of years the bark of this tree has been used to treat pain and fever. White willow bark contains salicin, a compound which provided chemists with the model for acetyl salicyclic acid—better known as aspirin. White willow is similar to aspirin in activity, but is weaker. Unlike aspirin which can cause stomach irritation, white willow also contains tannins, which aid in digestion.

THE RIGHT AMOUNT White willow is available in capsules

at health food shops. Take one to two capsules every three to four hours as needed.

POSSIBLE BENEFITS

Arthritis. Arthritis, which literally means inflammation of a joint, is a common ailment, especially among older women. There are many different forms and symptoms may vary, but typical symptoms include aches and pains in joints and connective tissue throughout the body. Aspirin and other anti-inflammatory medications are prescribed as the first line of defence against this disease. Good as these drugs may be, many have some very unpleasant and potentially dangerous side effects, including gastrointestinal distress and bleeding. For many people, white willow bark works as well as aspirin in controlling pain, but without the side effects.

PERSONAL ADVICE   Herbal medications may take longer to work than stronger drugs. Use this herb for two weeks to see if it helps control your symptoms.

WILD YAM

FACTS   Wild yam, often touted as the hot anti-ageing herb of the future, has an interesting past. For generations, southern blacks have used the root of this plant to treat rheumatoid arthritis and colic. Female herbalists have routinely prescribed it for menstrual disorders including premenstrual syndrome (PMS) and threatened miscarriage. In 1943 wild yam attracted the attention of mainstream medicine when a scientist extracted from it the female hormone progesterone—indeed, until 1970, this plant was the sole source of progesterone used in birth control pills. Today the herb is primarily used to treat two conditions associated with ageing: menopause and arthritis.

THE RIGHT AMOUNT   Wild yam is available in capsule form at health food shops. Take one capsule up to three times daily.

POSSIBLE BENEFITS

Rheumatoid Arthritis. Animal studies have confirmed that the steroidal saponins in wild yam have an anti-inflammatory effect and therefore may be useful in treating the pain and stiffness associated with a flare-up of rheumatoid arthritis.

Menopause. Wild yam is believed to regulate hormonal fluctuations that can cause unpleasant menopausal symptoms such as hot flushes, fatigue and vaginal dryness. This herb is often included in herbal formulae designed to relieve menopausal symptoms.

YOHIMBE

FACTS Since ancient times, different herbs and potions have been touted as aphrodisiacs. Few of these have withstood serious scientific scrutiny, with the exception of yohimbe. A compound extracted from the bark of the African yohimbe tree is a proven aphrodisiac that works well for many men. In fact, it is even prescribed by doctors under the generic name yohimbine or yohimbine hydrochloride to treat cases of male impotency.

THE RIGHT AMOUNT Yohimbine is available only on prescription and can only be used under the supervision of a doctor. If you are a man suffering from impotency, ask your doctor about this drug.

A weaker form of the drug is sold under the name yohimbe at many health food shops and herb shops. Yohimbe is available without prescription, but it is not as effective as yohimbine. It is often included in male potency formulae with other so-called aphrodisiacs.

CAUTION High doses of yohimbe can cause serious side effects in some cases. Yohimbe can lower blood pressure, and should not be used by people with hypotension. Yohimbe should not be used by people with medical problems unless under the supervision of a doctor.

POSSIBLE BENEFITS

Impotency. Impotency is a widespread problem for men over 40. In a recent study that appeared in the *Journal of Urology*, of 1,300 men between the ages of 40 and 70, at least half of those questioned claimed to have had trouble keeping an erection within the previous six months. Animal and human studies have shown that, in many cases, impotency caused by either psychological or physical problems can be successfully treated with prescription strength yohimbine. For example, in one Canadian study, 48 men were given either a placebo or yohimbine over a ten-week period. Of those taking the yohimbine, 46 per cent reported a positive response.

ZINC

FACTS In the not too distant future, a whole population of ageing baby-boomers may view this common mineral with new respect. In the body zinc performs many vital roles involving cell division, growth and repair—all of which tend to slow down with age. Men in particular may become interested in zinc, for there is a heavy concentration of it in the male prostate gland and many people, myself included, suspect that it may help to prevent prostate problems in older men. Last but not least, recent studies suggest that zinc may be an immune booster, and may even help to preserve vision in the elderly.

Marginal zinc deficiency is widespread among people of all ages, but especially among older adults, few of whom consume as much as they should.

Good sources of zinc include oysters, pork, liver, eggs, brewer's yeast, milk, beans, wheatgerm and pumpkin seeds.

THE RIGHT AMOUNT The RDA is 15 mg. Zinc is available in multivitamin and multimineral preparations. (Zinc gluconate and zinc picolinate appear to be the most easily tolerated.) Supplements range from 10 to 50 mg daily and I do not recommend exceeding 50 mg. Very high doses of zinc (over 150 mg) may actually depress the immune system and may also impair copper absorption.

POSSIBLE BENEFITS

Immune Enhancer. Several studies have been done on the role of zinc deficiency in the immune function of older people. One recent study showed that zinc supplements (220 mg twice daily for one month) increased the level of T-cells in people over 70. (T-cells help fight infection.)

Cold Fighter. Move over vitamin C—zinc may be a more potent cold fighter. In a study, 73 Dartmouth College students with colds were given zinc lozenges (zinc-gluconate-glycine) at the earliest stages of the illness. The lozenges reduced the duration of colds by more than 40 per cent (from an average of nine days to five days) and also greatly reduced the severity of symptoms. The students sucked two lozenges every two hours, up to eight per day. (Zinc lozenges should not be taken on an empty stomach because they can cause nausea.)

Vision. Macular degeneration, which causes a blur or blind spot in the field of vision, is a common malady of ageing which in some cases can be treated surgically. In one small study performed at Louisiana State University Medical Center, zinc supplements appeared to help control vision loss due to macular degeneration. In the study, 151 patients were given either 100 mg tablets of zinc twice daily or a placebo. Those who were given the zinc showed, in the words of the researchers, 'significantly less visual loss' than the placebo group. The National Eye Institute in Bethesda is embarking on a six-year study to determine the role nutrition and supplements such as zinc may play in the progression of eye diseases such as macular degeneration and cataracts. Perhaps by the twenty-first century we shall have some definitive answers.

Prostate. For years I have been recommending zinc supplements to men with prostate problems. There are heavy concentrations of zinc in the male prostate gland which manufactures prostatic fluid in which sperm cells are mixed to make semen. There is a great deal of anecdotal evidence supporting zinc's role in prostate health and male infertility although few scientific studies have been done. Recently, in the *Nutrition Action Healthletter* published by the American Center for Science in the Public

Interest, there was an interesting letter to the editor responding to an article in the newsletter which had stated that there was no scientific evidence linking zinc intake to prostate health. In the letter a Californian man pointed out that he was one of three brothers, all in their mid-sixties, one of whom was a regular user of zinc for 30 years, while the others were not. The two brothers who did not use zinc had developed enlarged prostates and even cancer—the zinc user had not. Coincidence? Maybe. But I have heard enough stories like this to make sure that I get sufficient zinc daily!

Up and Coming Supplements

Here are some potentially beneficial 'anti-ageing' supplements that are the focus of several research projects. I predict that you will be hearing a lot more about them in the near future.

DEHYDROEPIANDROSTERONE (DHEA)

Dehydroepiandrosterone (DHEA) is an adrenal hormone that is also found in Mexican yam. It is abundant in the young, but in middle age the supply begins to drop and by the age of 50 most people produce only one third of the DHEA that they did in their youth. By the time they are 60, DHEA levels are barely detectable.

Some researchers believe that the precipitous drop in DHEA makes people more vulnerable to many of the ailments that are often associated with old age, including two of the leading killers of both men and women—cancer and heart disease.

In one long-term study of men between the ages of 50 and 79, researchers found that those with the lowest levels of DHEA had the highest rate of heart disease. Other studies of normal men suggest that DHEA supplements can cut cholesterol, reduce body fat and increase muscle mass. Animal studies have shown that DHEA supplements can thwart the growth of artificially planted tumours in elderly mice and appear to extend their life

span. DHEA can also help improve memory, at least in laboratory mice, and may even make it easier to lose weight.

DHEA may sound like a wonder drug, but, like other forms
of hormone therapy, it has its downside. Studies show that
DHEA can cause the overproduction of sex hormones and liver
enlargement. In women, it can have an androgenic effect, which
means it may produce some unwanted side effects such as a
growth spurt in facial hair. However, researchers are developing
a 'safer' form of DHEA that should greatly reduce any risks.
Human studies are being conducted to determine what levels of
supplemental DHEA are safe for humans, and whether DHEA
is truly a life extender. Dr Arthur Schwartz, a biologist at Temple
University and a leading authority on DHEA, advises people to
avoid supplements until some of these questions are answered.

Wild yams are a natural source of DHEA, or take one to three
capsules daily.

HUMAN GROWTH HORMONE

Human growth hormone is released by the pituitary gland until
the age of 30 and is closely related to the stages of development.
Levels of growth hormone are high in the foetus, decline during
early childhood and surge again during adolescence. (Interestingly enough, the greatest amount of growth hormone is released
just before deep sleep, which could explain why adolescents
seem to need so much sleep.) After the age of 30, however, the
levels of the hormone sharply decline and in some older people
production seems to shut down altogether. As the level declines,
so does body function: low levels of growth hormone have been
associated with a drop in muscle mass, an increase in body
fat, diminished immunologic response, loss of appetite, and a
reduction in kidney function. Some researchers have speculated
that supplementing growth hormone in ageing people may
reverse some of these negative effects.

In 1990 Dr Daniel Rudman of the Medical College of Wisconsin and the Milwaukee VA Medical Center assembled 21
healthy men, aged 61–81, with one thing in common—
unusually low levels of growth hormone. Twelve of the subjects

received growth hormone injections over a six-month period; nine did not. Those who received the injections had a 14 per cent reduction in body fat and a nine per cent increase in muscle mass. Many of the subjects on hormone claimed that they felt better than they had for years, and growth hormone was quickly lauded as the 'fountain of youth'. Once the hormone was discontinued, however, the subjects quickly returned to their former state.

So why aren't we all taking growth hormone pills? Most scientists agree that more research needs to be done before the hormone can be used by the general population. It has some potentially hazardous side effects including cancer, arthritis, carpal tunnel syndrome and enlargement of the head, and it can also cause swelling and headaches, even at low levels. Several American studies on growth hormone are being funded to determine whether it works as well as it appears to do, whether it can be used safely and the optimum dose.

RU-486

RU-486 or mifepristine has gained notoriety as the so-called 'abortion pill'. The drug works by blocking key hormones necessary to sustain a pregnancy, including progesterone and stress hormones known as glucocorticoids. Many researchers worldwide believe that it may prove to be a real life-saver.

One French study showed that RU-486 shrank tumours in 25 per cent of women with advanced breast cancers. Progesterone can stimulate the growth of tumours, so any drug that can block the action of progesterone may also help prevent the growth of tumours. More studies are being done in the United States and elsewhere to determine whether RU-486 could be used in the treatment or prevention of breast cancer.

Other studies suggest that RU-486 may have broader application as a general anti-ageing drug. For example, in one study sponsored by the American National Institute of Child Health and Human Development, RU-486 was an effective treatment for Cushing's syndrome in six out of ten children given the drug. This study caught the eye of longevity researchers, primarily because the symptoms of Cushing's syndrome (which include a rapid decline in immunity, osteoporosis and loss of muscle) closely resemble a speeded up version of the ageing process. Research is under way investigating RU-486 as a treatment for osteoporosis, high blood pressure and adult-onset diabetes, among other maladies associated with ageing.

Words of Wisdom

Want to live to be 105? Follow the advice of the Delany sisters, authors of *Having Our Say: The Delany Sisters' First 100 Years*. At the time of writing, Sarah Delany is 105 and her sister Elizabeth (Bessie) Delany is 103. According to the Delanys, the secret of their longevity is a combination of diet and exercise. They do yoga exercises daily, and eat a clove of garlic chopped up and swallowed whole every morning with a teaspoonful of cod liver oil. In addition, they say, 'We eat as many as seven different vegetables. Plus lots of fresh fruits. And we take vitamin supplements: vitamin A, B complex, C,D,E, and minerals, too, like zinc. And Bessie takes tyrosine when she's a little blue.'

Chapter 3

Staying Well: A Guide to Preventing the Common Ailments of Ageing

In this chapter are listed the ailments that often affect older adults, and ways in which they can be prevented or treated without recourse to drug treatments. I believe that many of the drugs that are routinely prescribed for older people are not designed for an ageing body and often interact badly with other medications. Many of the problems commonly associated with the elderly, such as dizziness, confusion and weakness are caused by the very medication that is supposed to make them healthy! In my opinion, many of the ailments that the elderly are commonly treated for could easily be managed through natural alternatives, such as herbs, diet and changes in lifestyle.

People of any age should be wary of taking pills indiscriminately, but this is particularly true for people 50-plus. As we age, our bodies react differently to drugs. An impaired digestive system can interfere with drug absorption and a slowing down of liver and kidney function may lead to problems with breaking down and eliminating a drug, which can cause a toxic build-up. Memory or vision problems, or other physical ailments, could also be affected by medication. It is therefore vital for older people to be very wary of taking any medication without asking specific questions:

- What is this medication for?

- Can this medication interact with any other medication that I am taking?
- Do I have any other medical problem that could be adversely affected by this medication?
- Are you giving me the lowest possible dose?
- Is this medication safe and effective for a person my age?
- What are the side effects?
- Should I discontinue the drug, or reduce the dose, if I experience any side effects?
- Are there any alternatives to this medication?
- Do I take this drug with food or on an empty stomach?

It is my hope that a healthy lifestyle can eliminate the need for drugs. However, I recognise that it is sometimes necessary to take medication, and the right medication, at the right time, can indeed be a life-saver. As a pharmacist, however, I believe that no more than three drugs should be taken simultaneously, in order to avoid interactions or side effects, and that includes over-the-counter medications. If you must take several drugs simultaneously, be sure that you are being closely monitored by your doctor, and if you experience any difficulties with medicine, you should notify your doctor immediately.

In this chapter I recommend natural alternatives to conventional drugs, but if you are at present taking any prescription medications, do not discontinue them for any reason without first consulting your doctor. Do not substitute these natural alternatives for your medication unless you are under the supervision of a doctor or natural healer.

ALZHEIMER'S DISEASE

FACTS Alzheimer's disease is an irreversible form of dementia characterised by the slow but steady destruction of key areas in the brain that control reasoning and memory. Symptoms include memory loss, the inability to speak and difficulty in processing information. In most cases it is a late onset disease, affecting people increasingly from their late sixties onwards, but a few cases occur among people as young as 40.

Although we are quick to label any form of senility as Alzheimer's disease, there are many different types of dementia which can affect the elderly and can be caused by a wide range of factors including over-medication, stroke, poor blood flow to the brain and even depression. In contrast, Alzheimer's is marked by specific brain abnormalities—clusters of injured brain cells called plaques—which are believed to be responsible for the loss of memory and other behavioural deviations. The cause of the disease is still unknown, although it appears to be linked to certain genes. According to researchers at Duke University in North Carolina, people who inherit a gene that is responsible for producing a protein called Apo-E4 are four times more likely to develop Alzheimer's late in life, and if they inherit the gene from both parents, the risk is doubled. (In addition, these people do not produce enough of two other proteins, Apo-E2 and Apo-E3.) However, not everyone who has these genes will get Alzheimer's, and not everyone with Alzheimer's has these genes. Other researchers believe that the culprit is actually a protein called beta amyloid peptide that lies at the centre of the brain plaques. They suspect that this protein could be responsible for destroying brain cells.

There is no cure for Alzheimer's and, to date, drug treatments have been disappointing. However, there is strong evidence that simple steps can be taken to delay the onset of Alzheimer's, perhaps even indefinitely, or to lessen the severity of the symptoms.

Recommendations

Use it or Lose It: Many studies have shown that people with the highest level of education have the lowest rates of Alzheimer's disease. These studies were initially chalked up to the fact that better educated people tend to be more affluent, and more affluent people tend to take better care of themselves. However, recent research into the inner workings of the brain show that a lifetime of intellectual stimulation may have a far more profound effect. A child's brain is constantly producing new brain cells, but as we age production begins to fall off. Until recently, scientists believed that the mature brain followed a steady course of decline, but animal experiments have proved this theory wrong.

Studies on rats have shown that learning new tasks can actually stimulate the production of dendrites, threadlike appendages at the end of brain cells, called neurons, which help cells communicate with each other. The growth of dendrites did not occur only in young animals, as might be expected, but surprisingly, in older animals as well. Scientists speculate that human adults who are constantly challenged by intellectual pursuits may actually be building a bigger store of dendrites than those who are not faced with intellectual challenges. It is possible that when people with a reserve of dendrites develop Alzheimer's, which slowly destroys a portion of their brains, they may not experience as severe symptoms as people with less education and, presumably, fewer dendrites.

I'm not suggesting that anyone who has not attained a Ph.D. will get Alzheimer's disease. Education is not just about degrees, it's about staying interested in the world, learning new skills and accepting new challenges at any age. Make a concerted effort to 'grow your dendrites'—study a new subject, learn a new language, take up a new sport, or try your hand at painting or sculpting.

Limit Your Exposure to Aluminium. Some studies have shown high concentrations of aluminium—up to 50 times higher than normal—in some parts of the brains of Alzheimer's patients. This has led some scientists to speculate that aluminium, one of the most abundant metals on earth, may in some way be responsible for causing this disease. However, many researchers dismiss the aluminium connection, citing as evidence studies which show that people who live in areas with high levels of aluminium in their water supply do not suffer a higher rate of Alzheimer's than usual. Critics of the aluminium hypothesis also point out that half of all cookware used is made with aluminium and that if aluminium caused Alzheimer's, the disease would be more prevalent than it is.

Frankly, nobody knows what link, if any, exists between aluminium and Alzheimer's disease. The higher levels of aluminium found in some studies may simply be a result of the disease, not the cause. Nevertheless, I advise people to err on the side of caution. While it is impossible to avoid aluminium altogether—it is present in natural sources such as fruits and vegetables and small amounts may leach from aluminium cookware into food—it is possible to avoid ingesting high doses of the metal. For example, many commonly used over-the-counter drugs such as antacids and buffered aspirin are high in aluminium. If you are a regular user of either of these products, you could be ingesting up to 5000 mg of aluminium daily! Many deodorants are also high in aluminium—aerosol antiperspirants may be particularly bad because anything inhaled through the nasal passages is more readily absorbed by the brain. (Fortunately there are some excellent herbal deodorants sold in health food shops that do not contain aluminium.) Until we know for certain that aluminium is harmless, I recommend avoiding products with a high aluminium content.

L-carnitine. L-carnitine (see p. 78) is a non-protein amino acid that is found in heart and skeletal muscle. Its primary job is to carry activated fatty acids across the mitochondria (the so-called 'powerhouse' of the cell) providing heart and skeletal cells with energy. The brain tissue of mammals is a rich source of carnitine and some studies suggest that L-carnitine may be effective in slowing down the progression of Alzheimer's disease. Several European studies have reported that a daily supplement of L-carnitine (about 2g daily) can slow the mental deterioration typical of this disease (dietary intakes of L-carnitine average 100–300 mg daily). Although American researchers did not report good results from a major trial testing L-carnitine on Alzheimer's patients, since it is also excellent for the heart I see no reason not to use it.

Control Stress. Learning how to cope with stress, and getting help when you are feeling overwhelmed, may be the best preventative medicine against Alzheimer's. Several studies have shown that chronic stress can hamper the performance of cells in key parts of the brain, resulting in Alzheimer's-type symptoms such as memory loss and impaired mental capabilities. The damage occurs in the hippocampus, the portion of the brain essential for memory and learning. In animal studies, researchers have proved that prolonged stress can increase the signs of ageing in the brain, and many suspect that the same may be true for humans. During stressful situations, people produce cortisol, a stress hormone which revs the body up, giving them the physical and mental stamina to withstand the extra pressure. Researchers at McGill University recently found that people with higher levels of stress hormones in their blood did not perform as well in tests of attention and memory as those with lower levels. In fact, older people with lower levels of stress hormones fared just as well as young people in cognitive tests, while those with the higher stress hormone levels got scores up to 50 per cent lower.

Some researchers believe that people become more susceptible to stress hormones as they age. In some cases, people may produce too much stress hormone, which could cause damage to brain cells. Interestingly, stress hormone levels have been found to be higher and more difficult to control in Alzheimer's patients.

A Word about Oestrogen. Some studies have found that hormone replacement therapy may help prevent Alzheimer's disease in women. For example, researchers at the University of Southern California found that women who take hormone replacement therapy after menopause cut their risk of getting Alzheimer's disease by more than 40 per cent and, if they do get it, have much less severe symptoms. Other studies have shown that oestrogen can increase the growth of dendrites and trigger the production of choline acetyltransferase, an enzyme that helps carry signals among neurons. However, before taking oestrogen, keep in mind that another major California study has found that oestrogen has little, if any, effect on the incidence or course of Alzheimer's. Moreover, hormone replacement therapy is not without risk—women who take oestrogen increase the risk of getting cancers of the breast and uterus. Oestrogen can also be dangerous for women with certain medical conditions, including high blood pressure, clotting problems and migraine headaches.

Garlic. French researchers recently reported that aged garlic extract appeared to slow down brain deterioration in aged laboratory rats with an Alzheimer's type disease. The garlic also normalised the brain's serotonin system—if the serotinin system malfunctions, it can cause depression. Although we do not know whether garlic will work as well on human brains, I feel that since it offers so many other benefits, it is wise to include it in your daily diet or to take a garlic supplement.

ARTHRITIS

Arthritis, which literally means the inflammation of a joint, is a general term used to describe about 125 different conditions. The term encompasses a wide range of ailments ranging from osteoarthritis, the so-called 'wear and tear' arthritis associated with advanced age, to gout, a painful condition caused by high blood levels of uric acid, and lupus, an auto-immune disease that primarily affects women. Due to the ageing of the population, arthritis is a growing problem.

In this section I shall discuss the two most common forms of arthritis, osteoarthritis and rheumatoid arthritis.

Osteoarthritis

FACTS Also known as degenerative joint disease, osteoarthritis usually strikes after the age of 45 and is characterised by swollen joints, achiness, and stiffness or pain in the hands, spine, hips or knees. It is caused by a gradual wearing away of the cartilage, the spongelike material that cushions the ends of the bones, preventing them from rubbing together. In some cases, an injury to a bone or joint will cause osteoarthritis changes.

Bone X-rays of most people over 50 will show some signs of osteoarthritis, and although it can cause some discomfort it is rarely crippling. Indeed, researchers suspect that people with severe osteoarthritis may have a genetic form of the disease. There is no cure for osteoarthritis—as yet we do not know how to stimulate the body to regenerate cartilage—and for most people aspirin, or its herbal counterpart, white willow bark, or acetaminophen may be all that is needed to control the occasional bouts of pain. However, there are several things that people can do to prevent osteoporosis from becoming a problem.

Recommendations

Watch Your Weight. The knee is typically the first area in the body to be affected by osteoarthritis which, in severe cases, can impair mobility. Numerous studies have shown that overweight people are at greater risk of developing arthritic knees than those of normal weight.

Exercise. This may be the best preventative medicine against developing arthritis. Researchers suspect that exercise may help to retain cartilage by increasing the flow of blood to knee joints and other crucial areas, which is necessary to nourish cells. Walking, swimming, cycling and rowing are excellent choices for most people because they move joints in a safe way. Sports such as tennis, squash and soccer, which require pivoting and sudden moves, may be riskier in terms of injury. Contrary to common belief, even a high impact aerobic exercise such as running may be beneficial (but only for people who do not yet have osteoarthritis). Researchers at Stanford University studied the knee X-rays of 50 men and women who ran for about three hours a week. Some members of the study decreased their activity while others increased or maintained their running time. At the end of two years, researchers found no problems in the X-rays of the most active group to suggest that running had worn down cartilage.

At one time, people with osteoarthritis were advised to avoid the stress and strain of exercise. We now know that this was quite the wrong advice. For example, in a study conducted at the Hospital for Special Surgery and Columbia University, researchers found that people with osteoarthritis of the knee, who followed a supervised walking programme, experienced improved mobility and decreased pain in contrast to those who remained inactive. However, osteoarthritis sufferers should beware of any activity that further stresses already vulnerable knees and ankle joints. Running, jogging and sports that require a lot of pivoting, such as skiing and tennis, may cause more harm than good. So what's left? According to researchers, the solution may lie in the Far East: T'ai Chi, a form of martial arts based on gentle, flowing movements, can provide a good

157

work-out without overworking the joints. For more information on safe ways to exercise, telephone or write to Arthritis Care (See Resources, p. 252).

Avoid Injuries. Warm up before exercising—warmed up joints are less likely to be injured. Stretching limbers up muscles and tendons and improves joint mobility—in other words, it primes you for your work-out. Join a keep-fit class at your local health club. Most importantly, don't overexert yourself if you are tired—that is likely to make you accident-prone.

Become Safety-conscious. A little forethought can help to avert common injuries such as slipping on ice in the winter or falling in the bath, which can damage cartilage and begin a downward spiral of pain and inactivity. Wear solid, low-heeled boots or shoes out of doors. Be sure that your bathroom is designed for safety—more falls occur in the bathroom than anywhere else in the house. Repair loose or broken steps or anything else around the house or workplace that could promote injury.

DIETARY TIPS Some people find that certain foods may aggravate their arthritis. Obviously, if you consistently feel worse after eating a particular food, try eliminating it from your diet and see if you improve. Some people may find the night-shade vegetables (potatoes, tomatoes, peppers and aubergines) to be irritating.

ANTIOXIDANTS Some researchers believe that degenerative diseases such as arthritis are caused by damage inflicted by free radicals, highly unstable oxygen molecules which can, among other things, promote premature ageing. A daily antioxidant supplement including vitamins and minerals such as beta-carotene, vitamins C and E and selenium may help to prevent or slow down arthritic changes.

HERBAL REMEDIES

Ashwaganda. Part of the traditional Indian system of medicine called Ayurveda, ashwaganda has been shown to reduce pain and stiffness caused by osteoarthritis. Ashwaganda is sold in health food shops in tea and capsule form.

Boswellin Cream. Also from the Ayurvedic healing tradition, this greaseless cream contains extracts of *Boswellia serrata* plant, vitamin E, capsaicin and methyl salicylate.

Cayenne Creams and Ointments. Creams and ointments containing cayenne pepper can help reduce pain by stimulating the production of endorphins, the body's own natural painkiller. Many are sold over the counter at chemists' and health food shops.

Liquorice. This herb stimulates the production of two steroids, cortisone and aldosterone, which can help relieve pain and inflammation (aldosterone raises blood pressure, so liquorice should not be used by people with high blood pressure). Liquorice is available in tea and capsule form.

Rheumatoid Arthritis

FACTS This condition causes painful inflammation in the joints and can result in severe disability. Unlike osteoarthritis (which is caused by the wearing away of cartilage) rheumatoid arthritis is characterised by a hitch in the immune system, causing it to attack the collagen which lines the membranes of the joint. No one knows the cause of rheumatoid arthritis, although some researchers suspect that an initial infection may be responsible for throwing the immune system off balance, which triggers the autoimmune reaction. There also appears to be a genetic tendency to develop the condition. Although it can strike young women, most cases occur between the ages of 40 and 60.

If you have rheumatoid arthritis, you should be under the care of a doctor or knowledgeable natural healer. There may not be a cure, but there are many treatments available today that can help relieve pain and discomfort. In addition to conventional treatments, which range from anti-inflammatory medications such as aspirin or ibuprofen to antibiotics and immunosuppressor drugs, here are some alternative treatments that may help.

Recommendations

Gamma Linolenic Acid (GLA). Evening primrose oil contains Gamma linolenic acid (GLA), also found in borage seed (starflower) oil, an omega-6 fatty acid which is similar to the omega-3 fatty acids found in fatty fish. Natural healers have long prescribed evening primrose oil to treat rheumatoid arthritis, and a recent study performed at the University of Pennsylvania found that a daily dose of 1.4 grams of GLA could significantly reduce symptoms such as pain and joint swelling. Capsules of evening primrose oil and starflower oil are available at chemists and health food shops.

Omega-3 Fatty Acids. Several studies have confirmed that many people with rheumatoid arthritis have shown improvement after taking supplements of omega-3 fatty acids. They contain compounds that can inhibit the inflammatory response in the body.

Chicken Cartilage. Chew some chicken bones! According to a study performed at Boston's Beth Israel Hospital, chicken cartilage protein can help relieve the symptoms of rheumatoid arthritis. In the study, one group of patients drank a daily solution made from chicken collagen in a glass of orange juice, while the other group drank a placebo. Out of the chicken collagen group, four patients went into complete remission, while the others had a significant reduction in symptoms. In the placebo group, however, none of the patients went into remission, although a small group (four out of 31) said they felt better, which researchers attributed to the 'placebo effect'.

DIETARY TIPS. There is some evidence that a low fat diet may help to relieve symptoms such as pain and stiffness. In a study conducted by Loma Linda University in California, rheumatoid arthritis patients were given instructions on diet and stress reduction several times weekly for a five-week period. The participants cut their daily calories by about 30 per cent, and reduced their fat intake to about ten per cent of their daily caloric intake. After three months, the group experienced a vast improvement in the amount of stiffness and discomfort.

Other studies have shown that arthritis sufferers who eat a

vegetarian diet can find relief from their discomfort. Researchers cannot say whether meat actually contributes to arthritic bouts, or whether it is the increased intake of fruits and vegetables that alleviates the symptoms.

Some rheumatoid arthritis patients have found that certain foods may trigger a bout, and studies confirm that patients often develop allergic reactions to many foods. According to recent research, rheumatoid patients often show signs of sensitivity to foods such as corn, wheat, bacon, oranges, milk and oats. Researchers are not sure, however, whether food sensitivities actually contribute to arthritis.

HERBAL REMEDIES

Horsetail. This herb contains minute quantities of gold, which may be effective against joint pain and stiffness. It is sold in tea and capsule form in health food shops.

Propolis. Found in honey, this substance blocks enzymes that produce prostaglandins, hormonelike substances that can cause pain and inflammation. It is sold in health food shops.

Turmeric. This herb, which is used in curry powders, is a natural anti-inflammatory.

Wild Yam. This herb contains steroidal compounds that have an anti-inflammatory effect. It is available in tea and capsule form, and is used in many herbal arthritis formulae.

Yucca. This native American herb is an old favourite for treating rheumatoid arthritis, and is sold in health food shops in tea and capsule form.

CATARACTS

FACTS   A cataract is a cloudy or opaque covering that grows over the lens of the eye and can cause partial or total blindness. In rare cases cataracts may be due to a genetic problem, but most are a result of cellular damage to the eye lens inflicted by ultraviolet light or oxidation. Cataracts are very common among older people—it is estimated that as many as 50 million people worldwide are cataract sufferers.

Recommendations

Cover Your Eyes. To protect against ultraviolet light, wear sunglasses out of doors, not just in the summer, but all year round. Be sure to buy sunglasses that specifically promise to block 99-to-100 per cent of UVA and UVB rays. Not all sunglasses are effective, so check with your optician to see which glasses are right for you. A hat with a wide brim can also block about 50 per cent of UV light (and can help prevent against wrinkles).

Needless to say, avoid unnecessary exposure to UV light, such as tanning salons (which may also promote skin cancer).

Eat Your Fruits and Vegetables. According to researchers at the Human Nutrition Research Center at Tufts University, older adults with cataracts reported eating significantly fewer servings of fruits and vegetables than those who were cataract free. In fact, those who ate fewer than 3.5 servings of fruits and vegetables daily had a five times greater risk of developing senile cataracts than people who ate more. This is not surprising, since other studies have shown that people with cataracts have lower blood levels of carotenoids and vitamin C, compounds which are abundant in fruits and vegetables.

Take Your Vitamins. Antioxidants, such as vitamin C, beta-carotene and vitamin E may help guard against oxidative damage that can lead to the formation of cataracts. For example, in one study performed at the USDA Human Nutrition Center at Tufts University, when vitamin C was added to the diets of guinea pigs, their eyes showed less oxidative damage after exposure to UV light than guinea pigs who were not given the vitamin.

Other vitamins and minerals may also play a role in preventing cataracts. In a landmark study conducted by the National Eye Institute and the Chinese Academy of Medicine in Beijing, researchers gave more than 2,100 Chinese adults (ages 45–74) in a malnourished population of Linxian either two centrum multivitamin and mineral tablets and 25,000 iu of

162

beta-carotene daily or a placebo. After five years, the vitamin takers were 43 per cent less likely to have nuclear cataracts (cataracts which form in the centre of the eye) than the placebo group.

In a second test, more than 3,200 Linxian residents were given 2.3 mg of riboflavin and 40 mg of niacin daily. After five years, those who had taken the vitamins were 50 per cent less likely to develop nuclear cataracts than those who had not. Researchers suggest that riboflavin may have helped prevent cataracts because it is involved in the production of glutathione, a potent antioxidant in the eye lens.

COLORECTAL CANCER

FACTS   Colorectal cancer (cancer of either the colon or the rectum) is a leading cause of cancer deaths. About ten per cent of all cases are genetic—geneticists have so far identified at least two genes that are believed to be responsible, and even more may be involved. However, most researchers believe that perhaps as many as 90 per cent of all colorectal cancers may be due to environmental factors such as diet and lifestyle. Although colorectal cancer is common in the West, it is rare in the Third World.

The warning signs include rectal bleeding, blood in the stool and a change in bowel habits. (If you experience any of these symptoms, consult your doctor.

Recommendations

Cut Down on Fat. A high fat diet can indirectly promote the growth of tumours in the colon. During digestion, fat stimulates the release of bile acids by the gall bladder. The fat and bile then travel through the small intestine to the colon. In the colon, the bile is converted into chemicals called secondary bile acids which, in time, can product cancerous changes in the colon. The less fat consumed, the smaller amount of bile that is produced, resulting in a smaller amount of potentially carcinogenic secondary bile acids.

Wheat Bran. Researchers have known for some time that a high fibre diet appears to protect against colon cancer. However, recent studies suggest that wheat bran may be one of the most potent protectors. A study conducted at the American Health Foundation in Valhalla, New York, compared the effects of different dietary fibres on 78 women. Every day for two months, each of the women ate three to four muffins containing either corn, oat or wheat bran (consuming about 30 grams of fibre daily.) At the end of the study, researchers measured the level of tumour-promoting enzymes and bile acids in the intestinal tracts of the volunteers and found that only the wheat bran decreased the concentration of these potentially hazardous compounds.

In another recent study at New York Hospital/Cornell Medical Center, 58 people with precancerous polyps were divided into two groups. One group was put on a high fibre diet rich in wheat bran cereal and the other group was given a low fibre cereal. Most of the people eating the wheat bran experienced a reduction in the size and number of their polyps. There was no change seen in those on the low fibre diet.

Eat Your Quota of Fruit and Vegetables. A major six-year study of the diets of more than 764,000 adults by the American National Cancer Institute and the American Cancer Society confirmed that those who consumed the least amount of fruit and vegetables were the most likely to go on to develop colon cancer.

Protease Inhibitors. Compounds found in legumes called protease inhibitors may help to prevent colon cancer. For example, soya beans contain a unique protease inhibitor—the Bowman–Birk Inhibitor (BBI)—which has been shown to stop the spread of many different forms of cancer, including colon cancer. When rats were fed a carcinogen known to induce colon cancer, adding BBI concentrate to their diet suppressed the formation of tumours in 100 per cent of the animals.

Indoles. Indoles are compounds found in cruciferous vegetables including Chinese cabbage, broccoli, cauliflower and Brussels sprouts. Some studies suggest that indoles may help prevent cancerous changes in the colon.

164

Aspirin. In a study, performed by the American Cancer Society, of more than 635,000 people, those who took aspirin were at significantly lower risk of dying from colon cancer—indeed, men and women who took aspirin at least 16 times a month were 40 per cent less likely to die from cancers of the digestive tract than those who did not. Talk to your doctor about whether or not you should take aspirin.

Calcium and Vitamin D. Several studies have found a link between low calcium/vitamin D consumption and an increased risk of colorectal cancer. A major 19-year population study of more than 25,000 people in Chicago found that those who had an average daily intake of 1200 mg of calcium had a 50 per cent reduced risk of the disease. Researchers suspect that calcium may bind with bile, thus preventing it from irritating the colon wall.

Exercise. A sedentary lifestyle has been linked to an increased risk of colorectal cancer. In one study, men who scored the lowest in terms of activity had nearly twice the risk of colorectal cancer of the most active men. Presumably, the same is true for women.

CONSTIPATION

FACTS Constipation is a very common problem among older adults. As we age, the digestive system slows down, making it harder to break down food and eliminate waste. Hormonal changes during menopause can also cause occasional bouts of constipation in some women, and prescription drugs such as diuretics, painkillers, tranquillisers and even antihistamines can actually promote constipation. However, very often diet and lifestyle are the main culprits, and making simple changes can help to keep you regular.

Recommendations

Exercise. I think that inactivity is one of the main reasons why older people (and many younger ones) suffer from constipation. Sitting at a desk all day, or sitting in your car, prevents your body from working well. You don't have to overdo it—a simple walking programme could make a real difference.

Water. Drinking eight to ten glasses of filtered water per day will help to increase intestinal motility and prevent constipation.

Increase Your Fibre. Insoluble fibre—the kind found in foods such as celery, wheat bran, legumes and most fruits and vegetables—softens and bulks waste to help move it more quickly through the colon, thus helping to prevent constipation. Try to eat between 20–30 grams of fibre daily. However, it may not always be easy to get enough fibre from food alone. I therefore recommend taking *psyllium* daily. Simply add a teaspoon of psyllium to water or juice, and follow with two glasses of water. (Psyllium can cause allergic reactions in some people, so if you know you are allergic to different foods, consult your doctor before using psyllium.)

To prevent bloating and wind, add more fibre to your diet slowly—if you have a low intake of fibre, don't shock your system by forcing it to cope with the whole 30 grams in one day. Give yourself time to get used to the new foods. If you have a bowel disorder, consult your doctor before adding fibre to your diet.

CORONARY ARTERY DISEASE

FACTS   When we talk about heart disease, we are really talking about coronary artery disease (CAD), a condition in which the arteries bringing blood to the heart become clogged or obstructed with a yellowish, waxy substance called plaque (the condition is known as atherosclerosis). If the arteries become too narrow the flow of blood and oxygen to the heart will become severely impaired, which can lead to a heart attack.

Some people are more prone to heart disease than others due to such factors as age, genetics or lifestyle. The risk of developing coronary artery disease increases with age—about 55 per cent of all heart attacks occur after the age of 55. Before that, men have a higher rate of heart disease, but women quickly catch up after menopause. Race seems to be another risk factor. In the United States, people of African origin have a higher rate of heart disease than whites. People with a parent or sibling who has had a heart attack before the age of 55 (65 for women) are automatically put in a higher risk group. And in addition to immutable risk factors such as sex, age and race, there are other, more controllable risk factors that are equally important, including smoking, obesity, sedentary lifestyle, diabetes, high blood pressure and high blood cholesterol levels. Few people are 'risk free'. But take heart—even if you have one or more risk factors, it does not mean that you are going to have a heart attack. Although you may have no control over your genes or your race, you can control many of the other risk factors, and by doing so can dramatically reduce the odds of developing coronary artery disease.

Recommendations

Caution If you have a heart condition or are taking medicine for a heart problem, do not use any herbs, drugs or supplements without first consulting your doctor or natural healer.

Up in Smoke. Up to 40 per cent of deaths from heart disease each year are believed to be due to smoking-related problems. Given the fact that smoking has also been associated with an increased risk of developing many different forms of cancer, by now even the most inveterate smoker knows that it is time to stop. Increasingly, however, it is also being claimed that second-hand smoke from someone else's cigarette—or 'passive' smoking—may inflict damage on your heart. Researchers at New York University Medical Center have shown that passive smoking can accelerate the formation of plaque deposits in the arteries of male chicks. According to the study, the smoke-exposed chicks had plaques that were significantly larger than in those that were not exposed. Although no one knows whether human arteries behave in quite the same way, it makes good sense to reduce your exposure to cigarette smoke.

Keep Your Temper. According to researchers at the US National Institute on Aging and the University of Maryland, angry, hostile people are at greater risk of developing heart disease, especially if 'they are arrogant, argumentative, surly, and rude'. My hunch is that these people are also carriers, inflicting damage on their families and anyone else they come in contact with. If you find yourself losing control, seek professional help.

Monitor Your Cholesterol. Blood cholesterol levels should be maintained at under 200 mg/dl. HDL or good cholesterol should be 35 or above. The LDL:HDL ratio should be 3:1 but should never dip below 4:1. For example, if your LDL is 120, then your HDL should be 40. Eating a diet in which less than 25 per cent of your daily calories is derived from fat will help maintain a low cholesterol. In addition, watch your intake of saturated fat (primarily from animal products) and polyunsaturated fat from foods such as margarine, which contain trans-fatty acids that can raise blood cholesterol levels.

Foods that are rich in fibre, including oat bran, psyllium and pectin which is found in grapefruit, can help lower total cholesterol.

Keep track of another type of blood lipid—triglycerides. Elevated levels of triglycerides are a risk factor for heart disease. Women should maintain triglyceride levels under 200 mg/dl and men should maintain levels under 400 mg/dl.

Boost Your HDLs. If your HDLs are low, there are some things that you can do to raise them:

- Exercise has been shown to raise HDLs, especially if you have been sedentary. A two-mile walk four to five times a week at a moderately brisk pace may accelerate your production of HDLs.
- A glass of red wine daily has been shown to raise HDLs.
- An onion a day can raise your HDLs.
- Niacin (100 mg daily) taken with chromium picolinate (600 mcg daily) can lower cholesterol and raise HDLs. (High doses of niacin can be toxic to your liver and should be taken only under the supervision of a doctor.)
- Eating four to five smaller meals frequently throughout the day instead of the usual 'three square meals' has been shown to lower cholesterol and increase HDLs.

Take Your Antioxidants. Several studies have shown that people who take antioxidant supplements have lower rates of heart disease than those who do not. Antioxidants such as vitamin C, beta-carotene, vitamin E and selenium help prevent the oxidation of LDL cholesterol, which is believed to contribute to the formation of plaque.

Many herbs, including basil, dill, mint, parsley and rosemary, are excellent sources of antioxidants.

Aspirin. A recent study of 22,000 male doctors showed that those who took 325 mg of aspirin daily (the amount in one adult aspirin) had 44 per cent fewer heart attacks than those who did not. Talk to your doctor or natural healer before using aspirin on a regular basis.

Cut Down on Sugar. The Western diet is high in sugary foods, and this factor may contribute to the high incidence of heart disease. According to a recent study, high levels of dietary fructose, a sweetener derived from corn which is a common ingredient in processed foods, can raise blood serum LDL levels. Ironically, many of the new low fat or fat-free baked products on the market include fructose. Consume these foods in moderation.

The Amazing Olive. People in Mediterranean countries eat a diet rich in monounsaturated fats (mostly from olive oil) and, not so coincidentally, have the lowest rates of heart disease in the world. Studies have shown that monounsaturated fats can reduce overall blood cholesterol, and specifically can cut LDL cholesterol.

Monounsaturated fats combined with vitamin E may be a particularly potent way to attack LDLs. Researchers from the University of California-San Diego, La Jolla, discovered that oleic acid (which is found in monounsaturated fat) and vitamin E prevented the oxidation of a particular type of LDL—the smallest, densest portion of the LDL particle. Studies have shown that the small, dense LDL is more susceptible to oxidative damage than the larger LDL particle. About one third of all men and 15 per cent of all women have LDLs that are predominantly small and dense, and thus may be at greater risk of

169

developing coronary heart disease. In the California study, 18 healthy volunteers (nine men and nine women, aged 22 to 61) were given 1,200 mg daily of vitamin E. Six of the 18 volunteers ate the normal American diet which is high in saturated fats, six ate a diet high in polyunsaturated fats, and six ate a diet high in oleic acids. Blood samples from the three groups showed that the rates of LDL oxidation for both dense and larger LDL particles were lowest in the oleic-enriched group.

Omega-3 Fatty Acids. Found in fatty fish, omega-3 fatty acids have been shown to decrease blood cholesterol and triglycerides. They can also help prevent blood clots. Good sources include mackerel, salmon, albacore tuna, herring and river trout. Fish oil capsules are available at health food shops.

HERBAL REMEDIES

Several herbs can help prevent heart disease:

Capsaicin from hot chillies can lower blood triglyceride levels. Pour on the hot sauce!

Gamma Linolenic Acid, which is found in starflower oil and evening primrose oil, is an effective cholesterol-lowering agent.

Ginger. Ginger can help prevent the formation of blood clots, which can lead to a heart attack.

Ginseng can help lower cholesterol.

Green Tea. Several animal studies confirm that compounds in green tea, called catechins, can lower cholesterol. Not so coincidentally, Japanese men have the lowest rate of heart disease in the world, and Japanese women have the second lowest rate (second only to France).

Hawthorn. This herb has been used for centuries in Europe to treat heart ailments. Hawthorn is rich in bioflavonoids, which can help strengthen tiny blood vessels called capillaries, thus improving the flow of blood throughout the body. Animal studies have shown that this herb can increase the contractility of the heart muscle, strengthening the heart's ability to pump blood. In Europe, hawthorn may be prescribed along with the drug digitalis to regulate the heartbeat.

Oriental Mushrooms. Reishi and shiitake mushrooms can lower cholesterol and prevent blood clots.

Turmeric. This spice, which is used in curry powder, is a natural blood thinner.

OTHER SUPPLEMENTS

Coenzyme Q-10 is found in every cell in the body, but as we age levels of this enzyme begin to fall off. Coenzyme Q-10 helps facilitate the process that provides energy to cells and improves the circulation of blood. In Japan it is used to treat angina, chest pain caused by a diminished blood supply due to coronary artery disease. Coenzyme Q-10 capsules and tablets are sold at health food shops. I recommend 30 mg daily.

L-carnitine is a non-protein amino acid that is found in the heart and skeletal muscle, and helps to carry fatty acids across the mitochondria of the cell, thus providing heart and skeletal cells with energy. Some researchers believe that a deficiency of this amino acid may increase the risk of having a heart attack. Studies have shown that L-carnitine can also lower cholesterol and triglyceride levels and raise HDLs. L-carnitine capsules are sold at health food shops. I recommend 1 gram (1000 mg) daily.

DIABETES

FACTS   Diabetes is a disease characterised by an excess amount of sugar in the blood and urine. Juvenile diabetes, which occurs during childhood, is caused by the failure of the pancreas to produce enough insulin, the hormone that breaks down glucose or sugar so that it can be utilised by body cells. Adult onset diabetes is somewhat different. In this case, the body produces enough insulin, but the insulin works less efficiently. The precise cause of diabetes is still unknown, but in some cases, it may be triggered by a viral infection. There also appears to be a strong genetic component.

171

Most people do not think of diabetes as a disease of ageing, but that is precisely what it is. Eighty-five per cent of all cases of diabetes occur in people aged 35 and older. If untreated, it can lead to serious complications including heart disease, kidney disease, stroke and severe circulatory problems. Many diabetics require insulin shots and/or medication that stimulates the production of insulin by the pancreas. However, many are treated solely through dietary regulation and the careful monitoring of blood and urine sugar. Women are twice as likely to develop diabetes as men, but there is strong evidence that a proper diet and lifestyle can prevent or delay the onset of the disease.

Recommendations

Keep in Trim. Obesity is a major risk factor for diabetes (as well as a host of other diseases including coronary artery disease, stroke and several forms of cancer). Insulin is produced by special cells in the pancreas called beta cells, which manufacture and store insulin until a rising blood sugar level signals to them to release them. Over time, however, beta cells begin to wear out. It stands to reason that people who consume large quantities of food, especially sugar, may be using up their life's supply of beta cells quicker than others who consume smaller amounts of food.

High Fibre. Fibre-rich foods help lower insulin needs. A diet rich in legumes, whole grains, fruits and vegetables may be your best defence against diabetes (and many other degenerative diseases).

Low Fat. A high fat diet appears to hasten the risk of developing diabetes. In one study performed at the University of Colorado Health Sciences Center in Denver, researchers tracked the progress of 123 people with impaired glucose tolerance, a condition which dramatically increases the risk of developing diabetes. The researchers found that those who ate the diets highest in fat were much more likely to develop diabetes than those who adhered to low fat diets. In addition, in subsequent blood tests, people eating the lowest amount of fat had normal blood sugar levels.

Monounsaturated Fat. Recent studies suggest that increasing your intake of monounsaturated fat (found in olive oil, canola oil and avocado) may help stabilise blood sugar levels. Substitute other forms of fat, such as saturated and polyunsaturated, with monounsaturates. Do not exceed 25 per cent of your daily calories in the form of any fat.

Exercise. A study performed at the Human Nutrition Research Center on Aging at Tufts showed that regular aerobic exercise can lower people's risk of diabetes. Researchers studied 18 older men and women who had above-normal glucose levels on a glucose tolerance test, which increased their risk of developing diabetes by ten-fold. After 12 weeks of cycling on an ergometer four days per week, the 18 volunteers had increased their blood glucose clearance by 11 per cent. The exercise also appeared to improve the ability of their cells to respond to insulin.

SUPPLEMENTS

Chromium. Animal studies have shown that chromium, a trace mineral, can help the body use insulin more efficiently so that less insulin is required to break down sugar. Human studies have confirmed that chromium can reduce blood sugar levels in people who have elevated blood sugar. Chromium is found in broccoli, cheese, brewer's yeast, shellfish and whole-wheat muffins. Chromium supplements are sold in health food shops. Take 200 mcg daily in the form of chromium picolinate.

Magnesium. Older people often become insulin resistant—that is, their insulin does not work as efficiently as it should. Insulin resistance increases the risk of developing diabetes. Studies show that magnesium supplements can help older people improve their ability to metabolise glucose.

Vitamin E. A recent Italian study showed that daily vitamin E supplements of 900 mg for four months helped people with adult onset diabetes use insulin more efficiently, thus helping to normalise blood sugar levels.

HERBAL REMEDIES

US Department of Agriculture researchers used a test-tube assay

173

of insulin activity to identify plants that might help prevent diabetes. Nine plants were found to improve insulin activity, including sage, lavender, bearberry (*Arctostaphylos uva-ursi*), hops and oregano. (All these herbs are available from health food shops or herbalists.) Other potential herbal remedies for diabetes include:

Cinnamon. In test-tube studies, this spice appeared significantly to increase the ability of insulin to metabolise glucose. Take one to three capsules daily or sprinkle one to two tablespoons of cinnamon on your cereal.

Fenugreek. Fenugreek seeds (used to flavour curry and chutney) contain many different compounds that can help prevent surges in blood sugar. Take one to three capsules daily.

Garlic. Sauté some garlic in that olive oil! Garlic contains an amino called S-allyl cysteine sulphoxide which, in animal studies, has been shown significantly to decrease blood sugar and cholesterol levels. Garlic is also available in tablet and capsule form. Follow the package directions.

Turmeric. The spice which gives curry its golden colour, turmeric has been shown in test-tube studies to enhance the activity of insulin. Take one to three capsules daily.

DIGESTIVE DISORDERS

FACTS As we age, our bodies produce less hydrochloric acid which is essential for the digestion of food, especially fibrous meats, vegetables and poultry. As a result, it is quite common for people of 50-plus to develop chronic indigestion, characterised by gas and bloating after eating. Typically, people with this problem self-medicate by taking over-the-counter antacids. However, that is precisely the wrong treatment since antacids actually reduce the amount of the acid and the problem keeps worsening. If you have chronic indigestion, first consult your doctor or natural healer for an accurate diagnosis: the symptoms might also be related to an ulcer or other medical problem. If your symptoms are due to a reduction in HCL, try the following natural remedies.

Recommendations

Eat Smaller Meals. Small, light meals are kinder on the digestion than large, heavy meals. Try to eat small amounts of lean meat, fish or poultry accompanied by lightly cooked vegetables.

Digestive Aids. There are several over-the-counter digestive aids sold in health food shops that may help break down food. *Bromelain* is an enzyme found in pineapple that can help digest food and absorb vitamins. It is often used with *papain*, an enzyme found in papaya that can help break down proteins. Both are sold at health food shops in chewable, tablet form. Chew one 500 mg tablet daily.

Betaine Hydrochloride (made from beets) can also help to get the digestive juices flowing. Take one to two 500 mg tablets with food up to three times daily.

Herbal Teas. Several herbal teas are excellent for digestion problems. Anise, fennel and peppermint teas (all sold in health food shops) are particularly soothing for an agitated stomach.

DIVERTICULOSIS

FACTS Diverticulosis is a condition characterised by the formation of tiny pouches or diverticula in the wall of the colon. Diverticulosis is rare among children and young adults, but quite common among people over 40. By the age of sixty, about half of all people have diverticulosis.

Diverticulosis appears to be a natural part of the ageing process and is not serious. However, in rare cases the diverticula can become inflamed, which can lead to intestinal obstruction. The more serious diverticulitis appears to be related to chronic constipation and straining during bowel movements.

Recommendations

Avoid Constipation. A diet rich in fruit, vegetables and whole grains is usually all it takes to maintain regular bowel habits. For more tips, see p. 165.

GALLSTONES

FACTS The gallbladder is a sac in which bile from the liver is stored. Bile is essential for proper digestion. Gallstones are solid masses that form in the gallbladder or bile ducts, which can cause inflammation and pain. Up to the age of 50, gallstones are more common among women than men, but at that time men are equally vulnerable. People with liver disease may be more prone to developing gallstones.

There are three types of gallstones: cholesterol stones, those consisting of pure bile, and stones that are mixtures of bile, cholesterol and calcium. In some cases gallstones can be dissolved with drugs, but if not, surgery may be required to remove them. Chronic gallbladder disease may result in the surgical removal of the gallbladder. However, through diet and supplements, many people can successfully maintain a healthy gallbladder.

Recommendations

Low Fat Diet. An excess amount of fat may result in the overproduction of bile by the liver, which could lead to the formation of gallstones.

Lecithin. Lecithin supplements may help to control cholesterol build-up and may help to prevent gallstones. It is sold in granule and capsule form at health food shops. Take between 500 and 1000 mg daily.

HERBAL REMEDIES

Dandelion. This herb (or weed depending on your point of view) enhances liver and gallbladder function and has traditionally been used by herbalists to treat ailments related to these organs. Interestingly, dandelion is a rich source of lecithin. Eat fresh dandelion in salads, or buy the capsules at health food shops. Take one to three capsules daily.

Turmeric. Studies performed in Germany and India show that this herb may help to prevent gallstones, probably by enhancing the action of the liver and gallbladder. Use this spice in cooking or take a 300 mg capsule up to three times daily.

GOUT

FACTS   Gout is a particularly painful form of arthritis caused by the accumulation of uric acid, a substance that is produced by the body from purines, compounds found in many different foods. Excess uric acid forms crystal-like deposits in joints—typically in the large joint of one or both big toes—which can lead to arthritic-type swelling and pain. Gout is much more common among men than women, but after menopause, women are at a higher risk of developing this disease.

Gout tends to run in families, but in some cases, the condition can be brought on by the use of diuretics and other drugs. Gout can be successfully treated with allopurinol which can control the rate at which the body produces uric acid. Other medications can speed up the rate at which the body disposes of uric acid in the urine. Although drug treatment has proved to be quite effective, eating too much of the wrong foods (and drinking too much of the wrong drinks) can still trigger a painful gout attack. If untreated, gout can cause permanent damage to the joints.

Recommendations

Watch Your Weight. Being overweight increases the odds of developing gout. Researchers at Johns Hopkins University tracked the health and weight of 1,200 medical students for thirty years. Those who had put on the most weight during early adulthood had a much higher incidence of gout than those who stayed trim.

Watch the Purines. Much of the misery of gout can be prevented by maintaining a sensible diet. People with gout should severely limit their intake of foods rich in purines, including mackerel, brains, anchovies, sardines, shrimps, scallops and sweetbreads. Talk to your doctor or natural healer about the right diet for you.

Watch the Booze. Alcoholic beverages, especially taken un-diluted on an empty stomach, can trigger an attack.

Do Drink the Water. Ten to twelve glasses of water daily can help flush the excess uric acid crystals out of the body.

HERBAL REMEDIES

Many herbs have been used to help relieve the symptoms of gout, including:

Burdock Root. This herb has been touted as a 'blood purifier' because it can help control uric acid levels. Burdock is available in tea or capsule form at health food shops.

Juniper Berries. Herbalists have used juniper berries to treat gout and the herb may help to prevent attacks by normalising levels of uric acid. (Ironically, juniper berries are also used to make gin.) Juniper berry extract and capsules are available at natural food stores.

GUM DISEASE

FACTS Although people are getting fewer cavities thanks to the addition of fluoride in the water supply, gum or periodontal problems, which can lead to the loss of teeth, are still very common. Many adults have bleeding gums (a sign of inflam-mation), and the majority of all elderly people have significant periodontal attachments in their mouths, often due to tooth loss. Gum disease is usually caused by the accumulation of bacterial plaque near the gum line, which can cause gums to become inflamed. If the gingivitis progresses, it can destroy connective tissue and bones supporting the teeth. However, tooth loss is not an inevitable part of ageing: in most cases, gum disease can be prevented and teeth can be spared.

Recommendations

Oral Hygiene. I have difficulty in believing that there are still people who are not flossing their teeth daily. It is one of the best ways to keep gum problems at bay.

Avoid Sugar. Sugar is the breeding ground for bacteria. Limit your sugar intake and, in particular, avoid washing your mouth with sugary drinks. Keep in mind that carbohydrate is converted into sugar in the mouth; brush or rinse your mouth after eating.

Drink Green Tea. Try washing your meals down with green tea! It contains a compound that has an antibacterial action against *Streptococcus mutans*, the bacterium responsible for tooth decay, which can lead to gum problems.

SUPPLEMENTS

Calcium and Vitamin D. Animal studies show that low calcium intake can result in loss of the bone supporting the teeth. Be sure to eat calcium-rich foods or to take a calcium/vitamin D supplement daily.

Folic Acid. In human studies, supplements of folic acid resulted in less inflammation of the gums in people with gingivitis. Take 400 mcg of folic acid daily. (Doses over 800 mcg may be toxic.)

Propolis. This by-product of honey is a rich source of bioflavonoids, naturally occurring substances in food which may help to strengthen tiny blood vessels in the gums, thus helping to prevent injury. Take 500 mg capsules three times daily.

Vitamin C Complex (plus Bioflavonoids). Vitamin C is required for the formation of collagen in connective tissues, and is necessary for the repair and maintenance of all body tissues, including the gums. Vitamin C complex includes several bioflavonoids, including rutin, which has been shown to be especially beneficial for gums. Take 1000 mg daily of calcium ascorbate.

HAEMORRHOIDS

FACTS Haemorrhoids are varicose veins in the anus and rectum. (For a full explanation of varicose veins, see p. 198.) Symptoms include pain and light rectal bleeding. (If you have any rectal bleeding consult your doctor—it could be a sign of a gastrointestinal problem or even colon cancer.)

Chronic constipation, pregnancy or abdominal straining can cause haemorrhoids. In severe cases, surgery may be necessary. However, this is a problem that can usually be easily controlled through diet and the judicious use of supplements.

Recommendations

Avoid Spicy Foods. Hot pepper can aggravate existing haemorrhoids.

Fibre, Fibre, Fibre. The low-fibre diet typical of most people in Britain is the major cause of haemorrhoids. A diet rich in fruits, vegetables and whole grains can help keep your bowel functioning normally, which will prevent the kind of straining that can result in haemorrhoids.

Vitamin E. For quick relief, place some vitamin E oil on a cotton wool ball or Q-tip and apply to the affected area. (Some people are allergic to vitamin E oil. Be sure to try some oil on a small patch of skin and wait 24 hours. Watch for irritation or burning; if there is none, you can proceed with the treatment.)

HERBAL REMEDIES

Butcher's Broom. A salve made from this herb can be applied directly to haemorrhoids. Butcher's broom products are sold in health food shops.

Ginkgo. This herb helps to promote good circulation, which may help to prevent varicose veins, including haemorrhoids. Take one to three capsules daily.

HEARING LOSS

FACTS *Presbycusis*, the age-related decline in hearing, can begin at around the age of 20, when there is a gradual loss in high frequency hearing. The loss is usually so subtle that it is hardly noticeable. However, by the age of 60 there may be a noticeable loss of middle and low frequency hearing, making it more difficult to discern human speech. The extent of hearing loss largely depends on two factors: heredity and exposure to loud noises. However, atherosclerosis can also prevent the flow of blood and nutrients to the ear, which could also cause hearing loss.

Recommendations

Safeguarding Your Hearing. The best way to preserve your hearing is to avoid bombarding your ears with loud noises, which can actually cause permanent damage to the middle ear. The level of noise considered to be dangerous is 85–90 decibels—normal speech is usually 65–70 decibels. If you listen to loud music, work near loud machinery or use many common items such as a lawn mower or vacuum cleaner, you could be exposing yourself to decibel levels that are unsafe. Impulse noise, such as loud explosions from firearms or fireworks, are particularly dangerous. If you are in situations where you are exposed to loud noises, be sure to wear protective earplugs. They are sold by chemists and sporting goods stores.

HIGH BLOOD PRESSURE

FACTS When blood is pumped through the heart, it flows through the large arteries into smaller arteries or arterioles. The walls of the arterioles can expand or contract, thus regulating the blood flow. Blood pressure is measured by the force of blood against the arterial wall. The top number, called the systolic pressure, measures the pressure of the blood flow when the heart is beating. The bottom number, called the diastolic pressure, measures the pressure of the blood flow when the heart is at

181

rest. A normal adult blood pressure is around 120/80. High blood pressure is defined as a systolic pressure of 140 or above and a diastolic pressure of 90 or above. However, many studies show that a moderately elevated diastolic pressure (85 plus) may be a sign of a problem down the road.

Untreated high blood pressure is dangerous because it means that the heart is working harder than normal to pump blood, which can cause damage to the heart, arteries and kidneys. High blood pressure is a major risk factor for both heart attack and stroke.

In most cases, the cause of high blood pressure is a mystery. However, in about five per cent of all cases, the problem can be attributed to an underlying physical condition such as a congenital heart problem, kidney abnormality or tumour of the adrenal gland.

With many people in the West, blood pressure rises steadily with age. Men are likely to develop high blood pressure at younger ages than women, but by the age of 65 women are at greater risk than men. However, I want to stress that high blood pressure is not an inevitable part of ageing. In some parts of the world, blood pressure remains relatively stable from childhood through to old age. Many researchers believe that diet and lifestyle play a major role in helping to prevent high blood pressure.

There are numerous drugs that are prescribed to control high blood pressure. Although most work well, nearly all have some undesirable side effects ranging from excessive fatigue to impotency. However, there are many natural alternatives that may work just as well in helping to control high blood pressure, or even prevent it from happening in the first place. In many cases, simple changes in diet and lifestyle can also reduce the need for medication.

Recommendations

Lose Weight. Being overweight increases the risk of developing high blood pressure. Often, a loss in weight is accompanied by a reduction in blood pressure.

Watch the Salt. Many people are salt-sensitive—that is, excessive salt in their diet will cause an increase in blood pressure. The American Heart Association recommends limiting your salt intake to 2500 mg per day or 1000 mg per thousand calories. In order to achieve this goal, you should probably not add additional salt to your food and steer clear of restaurants that serve highly salted food.

Exercise. A regular exercise programme that requires aerobic activity, such as walking two miles daily, or swimming laps, can help maintain normal blood pressure. In some cases it can even lower blood pressure in people with high blood pressure.

Limit Alcohol. Drinking more than 50 ml daily of an alcoholic beverage can increase the risk of developing high blood pressure.

Load Up on the Fruit. According to a study performed at Harvard Medical School, eating a diet high in fruit fibre can help prevent high blood pressure. In their study, the researchers tracked the diets of more than 30,000 men and found that those who ate less than 12 grams of fruit fibre daily were 60 per cent more likely to develop high blood pressure. The researchers found that fruit fibre was more effective in preventing high blood pressure than fibre from grains. Keep in mind, it may not be just the fibre that has a protective effect. Fruit also contains many different compounds, including some that may help to lower blood pressure.

L-carnitine. Supplements of L-carnitine, a non-protein amino acid found in the heart and skeletal muscle, have been shown to improve the flow of blood to the heart and reduce blood pressure. L-carnitine is sold at health food shops.

MIND YOUR MINERALS

Calcium. A 13-year California study of more than 6,600 men and women found that people who consumed 1000 mg of calcium daily reduced their risk of developing high blood pressure by 20 per cent.

Magnesium. A recent Dutch study sponsored by the Netherlands Heart Foundation showed that magnesium supplements were effective in controlling high blood pressure in women with mildly high blood pressure who were not on other medication. Six months of magnesium supplementation reduced the systolic pressure by 2.7 and the diastolic pressure by 3.4. Good food sources of magnesium include legumes, green leafy vegetables, whole grains, bananas, low fat milk and apricots.

Potassium. Several studies have shown that potassium can help reduce blood pressure. In fact, in one study of 54 patients with high blood pressure who were on medication, half the group was given information on increasing their dietary intake of potassium, and the other half was told to continue with their normal diet. At the end of the study, those patients eating the most potassium-rich foods required the least amount of medication to control their blood pressure. In addition, the patients eating the potassium-rich diet felt better and had fewer symptoms. Good sources of potassium include white potato, dried apricots, banana, low fat yogurt and orange.

HERBAL REMEDIES

Astragalus. This herb, which is widely used in China, has been shown to lower blood pressure in animal studies. Astragalus capsules are available in health food shops and from herbalists.

Celery. Researchers at the University of Chicago discovered a compound in celery called 3-butylphthalide that can reduce high blood pressure in laboratory rats. Interestingly, celery is used by Oriental healers to treat high blood pressure.

Dong Quai. Studies have shown that this Chinese herb can lower blood pressure in both men and women. Dong quai is available at health food shops in tea and capsule form.

Hawthorn. Human and animal studies have shown that hawthorn, a well known cardiotonic, can reduce blood pressure during exertion. Hawthorn capsules and teas are sold at health food shops and by herbalists.

Motherwort. This herb is a mild sedative and can temporarily reduce blood pressure. It is available at health food shops and from herbalists.

Reishi mushroom. Compounds found in this delicious mush-room, which is widely used in Far Eastern cooking, can reduce high blood pressure. Reishi are available at Asian food shops and at better greengrocers, and in dried form from health food shops.

IMMUNE WEAKNESS

FACTS Immunity is a highly complex system involving the interaction of armies of blood cells and proteins which protect the body against micro-organisms (such as viruses and bacteria), other foreign substances and cancer cells. As we age, our immune system becomes less efficient, making us more vulnerable to disease. At one time it was believed that a weakened immune system was a natural part of the ageing process, but many researchers now suspect that nutritional deficiencies may be a major cause of immune problems in the elderly. Based on these studies, it appears that it may be possible to keep your immune system strong simply by maintaining adequate levels of crucial nutrients, and by using appropriate supplements.

Recommendations

Beta-carotene. Several studies have shown a higher incidence of various forms of cancer among people with low blood levels of beta-carotene. One explanation is that beta-carotene is an antioxidant, which means that it protects cells against damage by free radicals which can lead to cancer. However, recent studies suggest that beta-carotene has a specific effect on the immune system. In one important study, 21 HIV-positive patients were given very high doses of beta-carotene (180 mg or 300,000 iu) or a placebo. After four weeks the patients on the beta-carotene showed significant increases in several blood factors that fight infection, including T cells, an essential component of the body's defence system. Good sources of beta-carotene include apricots, cantaloupe, broccoli, sweet potatoes and pumpkin. Beta-carotene is also available in supplement form. Take up to 25,000 iu daily.

Vitamin B₂ (Riboflavin). Studies show that deficiencies in this B vitamin can decrease the number of T cells, which can impair immunity. Good food sources of riboflavin include low fat milk, yogurt, beef, fortified breads and cereals and green vegetables. It is also included in B-complex formulae and multivitamins. The RDA is between 1.3 mg and 1.8 mg.

Vitamin B₆ (Pyridoxine). Researchers have found that vitamin B₆ depletion in elderly people can result in a depressed immune system. Specifically, B₆ deficiency appears to impair the release of interleukin-2 and lymphocyte production, two important parts of the body's defence system. Good food sources include cantaloupe, cabbage, low fat milk and blackjack molasses. B₆ is included in many multivitamins and B-complex supplements. The RDA for B₆ is 2–2.2 mg. Do not exceed doses over 2000 mg.

Vitamin C (Ascorbic Acid). Several studies have shown that vitamin C can lessen the duration and severity of the common cold, attesting to its antiviral activity. It also appears to raise blood levels of glutathione, one of the most important anti-oxidants produced by the body, which also plays a role in immunity. The RDA for vitamin C is 60 mg. I recommend 1000 mg daily.

Vitamin E (Tocopherol). A recent study published in the *American Journal of Clinical Nutrition* showed that vitamin E supplements can enhance immune response in healthy people over 60. In this study, 32 healthy adults were given 800 mg of vitamin E for three days or a placebo. Those taking the vitamin E showed a dramatic boost in immune function, but not those taking the placebo. Good food sources of vitamin E include whole grains, vegetable oils, avocado, wheat germ and baked sweet potato. The RDA is 10 mg or 14.9 iu, but I recommend a supplement of 400 iu daily.

Glutathione. Glutathione is an antioxidant produced naturally in the body. A recent study sponsored by the Human Nutrition Research Center on Aging at Tufts University has shown that supplements of glutathione can dramatically improve immune function in older people. It not only enhanced the cell's ability to fight infection, but reduced inflammatory substances pro-

186

duced by cells. There is no RDA for glutathione. Take 50 mg capsules, one to two times daily.

Zinc. According to recent studies, as many as 30 per cent of all healthy people over 50 may be deficient in zinc, which could hamper immune function. Researchers at Wayne State University in Detroit gave 3 mg of zinc daily to 13 zinc-deficient men and women. After six months, the participants showed signs of improved immune function, notably higher blood levels of thymulin which is essential for the production of mature T cells. Good food sources include oysters, pumpkin seeds, lamb chops, brewer's yeast, poultry, fortified cereals, low fat milk and wheat germ. The RDA for zinc is 15 mg. To ensure an adequate amount of zinc, eat zinc-rich foods and take a supplement of 15–50 mg daily.

HERBAL REMEDIES

Astragalus. Researchers at Texas Medical Center found that a purified extract of astragalus can stimulate T cells in cancer patients with impaired immunity. In addition, other studies have shown that astragalus can increase the production of interferon, a protein in cells that fights against viruses. Astragalus is available in capsules at health food shops.

Echinacea. Several studies have shown that this herb can help the body ward off viral infections. Echinacea has been used to restore normal immune function in cancer patients receiving chemotherapy. It is a traditional native American treatment for colds and flu. Echinacea is sold in capsules and extract at health food shops.

Ligusticum (Osha). Called ligusticum in the Far East and osha in the West, this herb may boost the body's ability to fight against viruses. It was used by native Americans to treat viral, fungal and respiratory infections. Ligusticum or osha capsules and preparations are available at health food shops.

Shiitake Mushroom. Lentinen, a compound from shiitake mushrooms, may help activate the immune system and fight against tumour cells. The mushrooms are delicious to eat. Shiitake capsules are available at health food shops.

KIDNEY STONES

FACTS The kidneys are bean-shaped organs located just above the waist. Their primary job is to filter waste products from the blood. About ten per cent of all men and three per cent of all women (usually over 40) will develop kidney stones, a condition which can interfere with normal kidney function and may damage the kidneys.

Recommendations

Calcium. Most kidney stones are made of calcium and oxalate, a compound found in many plants such as spinach, tea, wheat bran, chocolate, nuts and rhubarb. At one time, people with a tendency to develop kidney stones were advised to avoid both calcium and oxalate. However, a recent study suggests that that advice was wrong. Calcium may actually help to prevent kidney stones. Researchers at Harvard School of Public Health studied the diet of more than 50,000 middle-aged men. Much to their surprise, they found that men who consumed the most calcium were 34 per cent less likely to develop kidney stones. The researchers concluded that the calcium might have somehow prevented the absorption of oxalate.

Watch Your Intake of Oxalates. Although you don't have to avoid foods high in oxalates, you should eat them only in moderation.

Potassium. Based on the same study of 50,000 men, researchers found that men who ate the most fruits and vegetables had the lowest rate of kidney stones. The researchers speculated that since fruits and vegetables are rich in potassium, this mineral may play a preventative role in the formation of kidney stones.

Increase Your Fluids. Be sure to drink eight to ten glasses of water or other non-alcoholic fluids daily. The Harvard School of Public Health study found that men who drank the most fluids had a 30 per cent reduction in risk of developing kidney stones.

Watch the Protein. A high protein diet has been associated with an increased risk of developing kidney stones.

MACULAR DEGENERATION

FACTS The macula is a part of the retina which is responsible for central vision—the kind of vision required for activities such as reading fine print, sewing or driving a car. Macular degeneration occurs when the macula is damaged, leaving a blind spot in the centre of the visual field. Macular degeneration is the leading cause of blindness among adults aged 50-plus. Laser surgery may help to stabilise vision, but recent studies suggest that vitamins and minerals may also be beneficial.

Recommendations

Eat Your Greens. A study performed at the Massachusetts Eye and Ear Infirmary in Boston suggests that a diet rich in spinach and other green leafy vegetables may help to prevent macular degeneration. The researchers compared the diets of 356 men and women (aged between 55 and 85 years), all of whom had advanced macular degeneration, with the diets of 520 men and women of the same age group, who had some other form of eye disease. The researchers found that the people who ate the most carotenoid-rich food had a 43 per cent lower risk of advanced macular degeneration than those eating food with the least carotenoids. In particular, two carotenoids, lutein and zeaxanthin, both found in spinach and spring greens, appeared to have the most potent protective effect. Interestingly enough, lutein and zeaxanthin form the yellow pigment in the macula of the eye. Although more studies must be done to determine whether these two carotenoids are truly effective against this disease, it makes good sense to include spinach and greens in your anti-ageing diet.

Zinc. Preliminary studies suggest that zinc supplements may help to prevent macular degeneration. Take 15–50 mg of zinc daily.

MEMORY LOSS

FACTS By the age of 60, most people will have experienced some decline in short-term memory and alertness. Ironically, long-term memory may work better than ever—in fact it may be easier to conjure up the name of a long-lost childhood friend than that of a recent acquaintance. Limited memory loss is not serious, and it is certainly not a symptom of Alzheimer's or senility. Nor is it inevitable that everyone will experience memory loss—indeed, some studies suggest that more than one quarter of all elderly people perform as well in memory tests as younger people. However, there are several reasons why many older people may find their memory beginning to wane. An older brain may not produce the same quantity or quality of chemicals involved in memory function. The blood supply to the brain could be hampered by atherosclerosis or other circulatory problems, and in some cases medication could be interfering with brain function. Nutritional deficiencies have also been implicated as a factor in memory loss among the elderly and there is evidence that emotions may play a role. Some studies have even shown that undue stress can trigger memory loss in the elderly, and that boredom and depression may interfere with brain function. However, diet and supplements may help to keep you alert and sharp.

Recommendations

Avoid High Blood Pressure. Older people with diastolic pressures over 90 (the bottom number) experience a decline in short-term memory loss, according to a study conducted at the University of Maine. The longer the person has had high blood pressure, the worse the memory loss. However, once the blood pressure is normalised, the memory loss will not deteriorate any further.

Vitamin B₁ (Thiamin). Studies have shown that low levels of this B vitamin can cause subtle changes in brain function among older people, which could contribute to memory loss. Good food sources of B_1 include brewer's yeast, unrefined cereal grains, mackerel, sunflower seeds, ham and peanuts. The RDA for B_1 is 1.0–1.5 mg for adults. Thiamin is added to most B-complex supplements and multivitamins.

Folic Acid. This B vitamin may prevent memory loss by helping to maintain normal levels of homocysteine, an amino acid found in the body. According to a recent study performed by the Agriculture Research Service of USDA, researchers found a strong correlation between high blood levels of homocysteine and the loss of memory and ability to learn that often accompanies depression in the elderly. Other studies have shown that folic acid supplements can normalise homocysteine levels in people with elevated levels. High levels of homocysteine have also been associated with an increased risk of heart disease. Good food sources include dark green leafy vegetables, sunflower seeds, wheat germ, liver and peanuts. The RDA for folic acid is 400 mcg. Supplements are available at health food shops.

Choline. The brain uses choline to make acetylcholine, a neurotransmitter that plays a role in memory function. As we age, we begin to produce less acetylcholine, or the acetylcholine that is produced is less efficient, which may be why many older people become forgetful. Some researchers believe that choline supplements can reverse this trend. Good food sources of choline include eggs, soya beans, cabbage, peanuts and cauliflower. I also recommend phosphatidyl choline, which is actually the active ingredient in lecithin. Take 1200 mg daily.

HERBAL REMEDIES

Club Moss Tea. Researchers at the Shanghai Institute of Materia Medica recently reported that they had isolated natural compounds in club moss called huperzine A and huperzine B which, according to animal tests, helped to improve learning, memory retrieval and memory retention. (Huperzine A appeared to be the more effective.) Huperzine raised acetylcholine levels by inhibiting acetylcholinesterase, an enzyme which breaks down acetylcholine. Acetylcholine is a chemical found in the brain, which is directly involved in memory and awareness. Drink one or two cups of brewed club moss tea daily. There are several different types of club moss—be sure that the tea is *Huperzia serrata*, and not some other species.

Ginkgo. Animal studies have shown that ginkgo increases the level of dopamine, which improves the body's ability to transmit information. Several human studies have shown that ginkgo can improve mental performance among elderly people who have shown deteriorating mental function. Other studies have shown that ginkgo also improves the blood flow to the brain (and to other vital organs), thus providing the brain with oxygen and nutrients needed to function at peak capacity. Ginkgo is available in most health food shops and even many chemists. I recommend a supplement called Ginkgo 24. Take 60 mg capsules or tablets two to three times daily.

SLEEP DISORDERS

FACTS Sleep disorders, ranging from insomnia to frequent night wakenings, are a major health problem, especially for people in their middle years and beyond. Many sleep disorders that affect people in their retirement begin during middle age— indeed, women over 40 are at particular risk of developing insomnia, often due to menopausal discomfort.

Sleep disorders can not only severely hamper someone's quality of life, but can have a profoundly negative effect on health. Several studies have shown that lack of sleep can impair memory and make it difficult to concentrate, handle stress and accomplish daily tasks. The fatigue caused by inadequate sleep can also make you more prone to accidents.

There are many myths about sleep, and one of the most prevalent is that the older you get, the less sleep you need. In reality, the experts say, if you needed eight hours of sleep at the age of 20, you still require the same amount at 40 or even 80. And although older people may experience different patterns of sleep than younger ones, such as more frequent night awakenings, very often some of the more severe symptoms, such as chronic insomnia, may be caused by a physical problem such as sleep apnoea or an emotional problem such as depression. It could even be something as simple as too much daytime napping or too little physical activity. However, as people age they may simply accept a bad night's sleep as a way of life. They shouldn't. There are many things that you can do that may help to restore a normal sleep pattern. However, if self help doesn't work, here are some tips to help you get a better night's sleep.

Recommendations

Watch the Stimulants. From early afternoon on, avoid drinking beverages containing caffeine which could keep you awake at night-time. Caffeinated beverages include coffee, tea and many colas and soft drinks. Chocolate also contains caffeine, so try to avoid eating chocolate late in the afternoon or evening.

The same goes for cigarettes. I personally think that cigarettes should be avoided all the time, but if you do smoke, keep in mind that nicotine is a powerful stimulant. Try not to smoke too close to bedtime.

Say No to a Nightcap. A shot of booze may lull you to sleep, but it also makes you more prone to night-time awakenings.

Get Enough Exercise, But Not Too Close to Bedtime. Daily exercise can leave you properly tired out at night. However it can have a stimulating effect that may last for several hours, so try to finish your exercise routine at least two to three hours prior to going to bed.

Sex. Sex is a natural relaxant that helps soothe the body and promote a good night's sleep. Orgasm triggers the release of chemicals by the brain that are natural pain relievers, which can help relieve any aches and pains that may be keeping you awake.

Avoid Sleeping Pills. Barbiturates can be habit-forming and can cause dangerous interactions with other medications. Although it may be tempting simply to take a pill, in my opinion the risks far outweigh any advantages. There are also many other remedies that work just as well, without any of the side effects.

Melatonin. Melatonin is a hormone produced by the pineal gland in the brain, which helps to regulate sleep/wake cycles.

Many scientists have suggested that a reduction in melatonin may be responsible for the disruption in sleep patterns experienced by some older people. Recently, researchers at Massachusetts Institute of Technology have shown that melatonin can quickly induce sleep in volunteers. I use melatonin when I travel to help adjust to different time zones. Take one to three (up to 9 mg) capsules or tablets about 1½ hours before bedtime. Occasional use is preferred.

HERBAL REMEDIES

Chamomile Tea. I always end my day with a cup of chamomile tea. It has a relaxing effect on the body and is a traditional cure for insomnia. Chamomile tea is widely available at supermarkets and health food shops. (Chamomile is a member of the daisy family, which also includes ragwort. If you are allergic to any members of the daisy family, avoid this herb.)

Hops. Hops, the flowers used to brew beer, can be sprinkled on your pillow for a good night's sleep. Dried hops are available at health food shops. They really work!

Lemon Balm. This pleasant-tasting herb has long been used to treat nervous tension and insomnia. It is available in tea form at health food shops. Drink one cup daily.

Peppermint. This herb has a soothing effect on the body and may help to promote sleep. It is also excellent for heartburn and stomach-ache, two conditions which can interfere with sleep. Peppermint tea is sold at supermarkets and health food shops. Drink one cup at night.]

Siberian Ginseng. Unlike other forms of ginseng which can cause sleeplessness in some people, Siberian ginseng (*Eleutherococcus senticosus*) is used by Chinese healers to treat insomnia. Siberian ginseng is sold by herbalists and health food shops in capsules, teas and extracts. Take one capsule up to three times daily or drink one to two cups of tea daily.

Skullcap. This herb is a traditional remedy for insomnia and muscle tension. It is available at health food shops and from herbalists as capsules and tea. Take one capsule up to three times daily, or drink one cup of tea daily, preferably towards evening.

Valerian. Herbal healers use valerian to treat insomnia due to anxiety-related problems. Valerian is sold by herbalists and in health food shops as capsules or tea. Take up to three capsules daily, or drink one cup of tea daily.

STROKE

FACTS   A stroke occurs when the brain is deprived of oxygen and nutrients due to the rupture or obstruction of the arteries supplying blood to the brain. Most strokes are caused by blood clots that form in the artery bringing blood to the brain, or lodge there from some other point in the body. A minority of strokes are caused when a blood vessel on the surface of the brain ruptures and bleeds, or when a defective artery in the brain bursts. The telltale signs of a stroke are sudden weakness or numbness in the face, arm or leg on one side of the body; loss or slurring of speech; difficulty understanding others; sudden and severe dizziness or headaches. Strokes can result in permanent disability. About ten per cent of all strokes are preceded by transient ischaemic attacks, so-called 'little strokes' in which the symptoms disappear within a short time.

The incidence of stroke is directly related to age and sex: men are three times more likely to suffer strokes than women. There is growing public awareness about symptoms and risk factors but, sadly, I still feel that many strokes that occur could have been prevented.

Recommendations

Watch Your Blood Pressure. High blood pressure is the major risk factor for stroke. For information on how to control your blood pressure, see p. 181.

Stub it out. If you smoke, you are twice as likely to have a stroke as a non-smoker.

Maintain Normal Cholesterol. People with coronary artery disease are at an increased risk of having a stroke. Having high cholesterol levels in your blood will increase the odds of developing coronary artery disease.

Watch the Scales. Being overweight can increase your risk of high blood pressure which, in turn, will increase your risk of stroke.

PROTECTIVE FOODS

Helpful Vegetables. A study of 87,000 female nurses showed that eating lots of carrots and spinach can significantly lower a woman's risk of stroke, and presumably a man's, too. Carrots and spinach are rich in antioxidants, including carotenoids, which may help prevent arteries from becoming clogged with cholesterol.

Citrus Fruits. Citrus contains coumarins, natural blood thinners which may help prevent the formation of clots.

Something Fishy. A landmark Dutch study shows that men who eat more than 20 grams of fish daily have a lower risk of stroke than those who eat less fish. However, don't go overboard on the fish: a previous study among Eskimos has shown that those who ate the most fatty fish (including mackerel, salmon, sardines and albacore tuna) had the greatest risk of haemorrhagic strokes. To be on the safe side, stick to two or three fish meals per week.

Garlic. The 'stinking rose', as it is sometimes called, contains a compound called ajoene, which is a natural blood thinner.

SUPPLEMENTS

Aspirin. Aspirin can prevent the formation of blood clots. Many doctors advise their patients to take a small dose (one baby aspirin) daily or every other day to prevent heart attack and stroke. (No one should take aspirin routinely unless under the supervision of a doctor or natural healer.)

Selenium. Studies have shown that people who live in areas with the lowest level of selenium in the soil have the highest rate of stroke. Be sure to eat selenium-rich foods, including garlic, onions, red grapes, broccoli, whole wheat and chicken. Selenium supplements are available at health food shops; selenium is often included in antioxidant formulae. (Doses of over 200 mcg daily may be toxic.)

Vitamin E. Many studies have documented vitamin E's ability to prevent blood clots, which can help prevent stroke. Good food sources include olive oil, whole grains, avocado, baked sweet potato and oatmeal. Vitamin E is available in supplement form at health food shops. Take 400–800 iu daily.

HERBAL REMEDIES

Ginkgo. This ancient herb improves circulation to the brain and can prevent the formation of blood clots. Ginkgo capsules are available at health food shops.

Ginger. Ginger prevents 'sticky blood'—that is, it prevents blood cells from sticking together to form clots. Ginger capsules and teas are available at health food shops. Ginger is widely used in Asian cuisines.

Ligusticum. Studies have shown that this Chinese herb can help resolve blood clots in patients who have had 'little strokes' and can help improve blood flow to the brain. Ligusticum is available in capsule or liquid form at health food shops and from herbalists.

TASTE LOSS

FACTS   As we age our senses of taste and smell begin to wane. By the age of 60, there is usually a noticeable decline in the ability to taste food, due to a reduction in the number of taste buds on the tongue. Although this loss is not a medical problem, it can lead to one if it results in a loss of interest in eating, which can lead to malnutrition.

Recommendations

Zinc. A daily supplement of 15–60 mg of zinc gluconate may help to wake up your taste buds.

Check Your Medication. Certain drugs can interfere with the ability to taste food. For example, aspirin can increase sensitivity to bitter flavours, and several other medications, including some antibiotics, can cause a lingering aftertaste that may mask the flavour of food. If you are taking medication, ask your doctor if it could be hindering your taste buds.

Try New Seasonings. Spice up your cuisine—and wake up your taste buds—with a wide variety of herbs and spices. Avoid using too much pepper because it can have a numbing effect on your taste buds.

Variety. Stimulate your taste buds by eating a variety of foods with a variety of textures.

VARICOSE VEINS

FACTS A vein is a blood vessel that carries blood back to the heart. (An artery is a blood vessel that carries blood away from the heart.) A series of valves helps to push blood through the veins, but as people age, the valves become less efficient and the skin supporting the veins can become less elastic. As a result, the veins may lose some of their tone so that blood starts to accumulate. After a time the veins may become distended and varicosities may form. Typically, the veins in the legs are most susceptible to becoming varicose, but other affected sites can includes the testes and the oesophagus. Varicose veins are not only unsightly, they can also be quite painful.

In some cases varicose veins are genetic, but pregnancy, prolonged standing or even excessive strain of the abdominal region can also cause varicosities. Women are four times more likely to develop varicose veins than men, which suggests that hormones may play a role.

In severe cases varicose veins can be surgically corrected.

However, there are some things you can do that may help to prevent the problem arising in the first place.

Recommendations

Keep Moving. Although prolonged standing on one spot may cause blood to pool in the legs, exercise can improve circulation. A brisk walk or jog can actually help push the blood through the veins, as well as tone up the leg muscles which, in turn, help the valves to work more efficiently.

Bioflavonoids. Rutin, a bioflavonoid, may help to prevent varicose veins by strengthening capillaries, which are tiny blood vessels. Bioflavonoid supplements are available at health food shops.

HERBAL REMEDIES

Ginkgo. This ancient herb is used to treat circulatory disorders, including varicose veins. It is rich in bioflavonoids, which may in part explain its beneficial effect on blood flow.

Butcher's Broom. In Europe this herb is a popular treatment for varicose veins and related disorders. It is available in capsules or as a salve which can be placed directly on the affected area.

Gotu-Kola. Also known as centella, this herb has been used to treat inflammation and swelling associated with varicose veins. It is available in capsules at health food shops.

Vitamin E. Vitamin E helps to circulate blood to your legs and other extremities. Take 800–1200 iu of the dry form.

Chapter 4

Just for Women

As more and more women enter their middle years, I am constantly asked about menopause, breast cancer and other health-related issues of particular concern to women. In this chapter I shall address some of these questions, and discuss how women can stay healthy and vigorous for their entire lives.

Sexual Health

FACTS Between the ages of 45 and 55, most women enter menopause, a time of life marked by profound hormonal changes. During this time, production of oestrogen by the ovaries begins to decline and menstruation becomes erratic, lighter and eventually slowly begins to taper off. Once menstruation stops the ovaries continue to produce oestrogen, but in much smaller quantities. The word 'menopause' actually refers to the last menstrual cycle, but the entire process can take several years.

The average age for menopause is 51, but heavy smokers can become menopausal up to ten years earlier, and light smokers up to three years earlier.

Menopause affects women in different ways. Many experience very few changes and suffer few of the unpleasant symptoms often associated with the 'change of life'. Others, however, may have a more difficult time adjusting to the sudden fluctuations in hormones.

Millions of women take synthetic hormones (hormone replacement therapy or HRT) to help cope with menopausal symptoms. Hormonal therapy is not without risk, as I shall discuss later in this chapter, and there are some tried and true natural alternatives that may ease some of the discomfort of menopause without any of the risk associated with HRT. Here are some common problems that women may experience during menopause, together with some natural remedies.

BLOATING

Hormonal changes in menopause can cause the retention of water, which can result in PMS-type bloating. For some women the bloating is mild, but for others it can be so severe that it is difficult for them to wear anything with a defined waist line. Here are some herbs that may help.

Recommendations

Alfalfa. Also rich in phyto-oestrogens, the leaves of the alfalfa plant are an excellent diuretic. You can toss fresh alfalfa sprouts in salad, or the dried herb is available in capsules or tea. Take 3–6 tablets daily or drink one cup of tea daily. *(Alfalfa can aggravate lupus, an autoimmune disorder, so if you have lupus or a lupus-like disease, do not use this herb.)*

Centella. Also known as gotu-kola, this herb is a mild diuretic and has also been used to treat depression, another problem which can occur during menopause. Centella is available in capsules. Take one capsule up to three times daily.

Dandelion. This plant, which is also rich in phyto-oestrogens, is one of the best natural diuretics. The dried herb is available in capsules and tea. Drink one cup of dandelion tea daily or take one capsule up to three times daily. Dandelion leaves can also be added to salads. Dandelion is abundant in potassium, a mineral which is often sapped from the body by synthetic diuretics.

Hawthorn. This herb is known as a cardiotonic because of its positive effects on the cardiovascular system; it is also a mild diuretic. It is available in capsules or tea. Take one capsule up to three times daily, or drink one to three cups of tea.

Other herbal diuretics include wild oregon grape or osha, burdock, nettle, chaparral, celery and asparagus.

201

CAUTION Many women use liquorice root to relieve some of the symptoms of menopause. However, liquorice can promote the retention of water and should not be used by women who are prone to bloating, or by those with high blood pressure.

DRY MOUTH

The drop in oestrogen may also result in less saliva production, which can create a dry, gritty feeling in the mouth.

Recommendations

Water. It seems obvious, but be sure to drink at least six to eight glasses of water daily. Sip water throughout the day to keep your mouth and teeth moist. Chewing sugar-free gum, or sucking sugar-free sweets may help.

Slippery Elm Bark. Cough drops made from this herb may also help to moisturise your mouth.

Synthetic Saliva Sprays. These sprays are sold over the counter and may also offer some relief.

Evening Primrose Oil. Two capsules taken up to three times daily can help this condition.

If all else fails, there are several prescription products available which promote saliva formation and may be helpful. Consult your doctor.

FATIGUE

During menopause it is not uncommon for women to complain of excessive fatigue which is most often due to hormonal changes. Some women may be woken at night by hot flushes, others may have difficulty in sleeping.

Recommendations

Suma. Many herbalists recommend the South American herb suma to treat fatigue. Also known as South American ginseng, this herb is widely available at health food shops. Take one to three capsules up to two times daily.

HOT FLUSHES

About fifty per cent of all women experience hot flushes during menopause. A hot flush is a sudden feeling of intense heat followed by sweating and sometimes chills. For some women a hot flush can be a temporary nuisance, but for others it may be debilitating. Hot flushes are caused by hormonal surges by the pituitary, which is trying to stimulate the production of oestrogen by the ovaries. Stimulants such as caffeine and alcohol (which is also a depressant) may promote hot flushes.

Recommendations

Many women have found that supplements of vitamin E (400–800 iu daily) and vitamin C (1000 mg daily) can help prevent hot flushes. There are also several herbs that may help:

Ginseng, a herb which is rich in a plant form of oestrogen, has been successfully used as a treatment by herbalists. Ginseng is available in tea and capsule form. Drink one to two cups of tea daily, or take one to three capsules. I recommend American or Siberian ginseng since panax ginseng, which is commonly used in the Far East, may be too stimulating for many people and could cause insomnia. In rare cases ginseng may cause vaginal bleeding. If you experience any irregular bleeding during menopause, consult your doctor or natural healer, and be sure to tell him or her if you are using ginseng. Ginseng should not be used by people with high blood pressure or irregular heart beats.

Dong Quai. This herb, which is highly prized in the Far East, is known as the female ginseng. It is mildly oestrogenic in action, and may help relieve hot flushes and also other menopausal symptoms.

Vitex. This herb is used to regulate hormonal balance. Unlike ginseng or dong quai, it is not oestrogenic in action and is a very popular menopause aid. Vitex is available in capsules and in 'change of life' herbal formulae for women. Take as directed.

Diet may also help. Interestingly enough, in Japan there is no word for 'hot flush', and its omission from the language reflects the fact that it is a rare symptom there. Japanese women eat a diet rich in soya foods such as tofu, tempeh and soya milk, all excellent sources of phyto-oestrogens, plant compounds which behave like oestrogen in the body. Researchers speculate that these plant oestrogens, although they are much weaker than real hormones, may help to relieve some of the symptoms of menopause that are caused by a decline in the production of natural oestrogen. Other foods that are rich in phyto-oestrogens include alfalfa, cherries, barley, apples, rye, potatoes, rice, wheat, yams and yeast.

Deep breathing may also provide relief from hot flushes. In a recent study of 33 menopausal women experiencing hot flushes, slow, deep, abdominal breathing appeared to cut the rate of occurrence by half. The researchers suspect that the deep breathing may lower the arousal of the central nervous system which usually occurs prior to a hot flush. Deep breathing can be used to prevent hot flushes, or to try to ward one off if you feel it coming on. Simply take slow, relaxed breaths for about 15 minutes. Be sure you are really breathing from your stomach— your abdomen should fill up with air. Do this exercise twice daily.

MOOD SWINGS

As in PMS, many women find that they experience mood swings, depression or irritability during menopause which are often caused by hormonal fluctuations.

Recommendations

The herbs usually given for menopause, including dong quai, vitex and ginseng, may help promote a feeling of energy and well-being. Also try these remedies:

Vitamin B₆. This vitamin is commonly used to treat depression or moodiness due to menopause. Take between 50 and 100 mg daily in supplement form. In rare cases, daily doses over 200 mg could be toxic.

Hops. This herb, which is rich in phyto-oestrogens, may help relax and soothe. It is especially good for women bothered by insomnia. Traditionally, people used to sprinkle hops with alcohol, put them in a pillowcase and sleep on it. Hop pillows can still be bought from herbalists, health food shops and country craft shops, but hops are also available in capsules. Take one to three daily.

Ginger. A cup of ginger tea is a nice pick-me-up.

VAGINAL DRYNESS

The drop in oestrogen can cause a thinning in the vaginal lining and a decline in vaginal lubrication. This can result in painful intercourse and makes the vagina more vulnerable to yeast and other infections.

Recommendations

Many women have found that vitamin E supplements (400 to 800 iu) can help prevent vaginal dryness. Here are some other things you can try:

Dong Quai. Many women rely on dong quai for this and other menopause-related problems. Take one capsule up to three times daily.

Wild Yam. This herb, a rich source of plant hormones, may help prevent vaginal dryness. It is available in capsules. Take one up to three times daily.

Vaginal Moisturisers. There are many over-the-counter products that can help lubricate the vagina. To avoid potential irritants, be sure to buy one that is unscented.

Pelvic Floor Exercises. These simple exercises can help promote circulation to the vaginal lining and maintain vaginal muscle tone. Squeeze your vaginal muscles—it should feel as if you are trying to stop urinating midstream—hold in your muscles tightly for about ten seconds, then release. Repeat this exercise for up to ten minutes twice daily.

YEAST AND URINARY TRACT INFECTIONS

The thinning of the vaginal and urethral lining makes women more prone to yeast and urinary tract infections.

Recommendations

Lactobacillus Acidophilus. This so-called 'friendly bacterium' found in yogurt may help prevent yeast infections. If yeast infections are a problem, eat two cartons of yogurt daily (which is also a terrific way to get calcium) or take two acidophilus capsules half an hour before or after meals, three times daily.

Cranberry Capsules. These may help to prevent urinary tract infections. Take two capsules up to three times daily or drink two glasses of unsweetened cranberry juice daily.

Uva-Ursi. This herb is commonly used to treat urinary tract infections in women and men. Take one capsule up to three times daily to relieve symptoms.

Breast Cancer

FACTS Breast cancer is a leading cause of cancer death among women. It is a very serious problem, but the oft-quoted figure that one out of nine women will get breast cancer is somewhat misleading. The risk of developing breast cancer increases dramatically with age: a 20-year-old woman has a significantly lower risk of getting breast cancer than a 40-year-old, and a 40-year-old woman has a significantly lower risk than a 60-year-old, and so on.

The incidence and mortality rate of breast cancer is much higher in Western Europe and the United States than it is in Asia or Africa. For example, American women are four times more likely to die from breast cancer than are Japanese women; yet when Japanese women emigrate to the United States, within one or two generations their mortality rate from breast cancer is equal to that of the native population. Researchers speculate that breast cancer may be caused by environmental factors such as diet or exposure to cancer-causing chemicals.

Genetics may also play a role in breast cancer, but it appears to be a small one. Only about six per cent of all cases of breast cancer are believed to be linked to heredity; which means that more than 90 per cent of all cases occur in women who have no previous family history of the disease.

Why is the rate of breast cancer so high in the Western world? Is there anything a woman can do to reduce her risk? Although we do not have all the answers, there is some compelling evidence that diet and lifestyle may help prevent breast cancer.

The Low-Down on Fat

One obvious difference between the Western world and countries in Asia and Africa is diet in general and fat in particular. Our diet contains nearly two to three times the amount of fat eaten in the developing countries. In particular, Westerners eat much more saturated fat, notably from dairy and animal products. In the human body, hormones are stored in fatty tissue. The female hormone oestrogen has been shown to trigger the growth of oestrogen-sensitive tumours in the breast and other parts of the body (more than half of all breast tumours are oestrogen-sensitive), so it is possible that a diet high in fat could result in more fat stores in the body, and higher levels of hormones. In addition, in menopausal women hormones produced by the adrenal gland are converted into oestrogen by fat

207

cells, which could explain why obesity is a risk factor for breast cancer among menopausal women.

Fat is also the storage site for many potentially dangerous carcinogens that we get from food and other sources, which may also spur the growth of tumours.

Epidemiological studies—that is, studies of large populations, have shown a definite link between the consumption of fat and a higher rate of breast cancer among men. For example, in the United States, Seventh Day Adventists, many of whom are vegetarians and consume less fat than the general population, have up to a 75 per cent reduced risk of dying of breast cancer. Animal studies have shown a direct correlation between a high fat diet and the growth of breast tumours, but human studies have been more ambiguous. A major study of nurses published in the American *Journal of the National Cancer Institute* showed that there was little difference between the fat intake of women who developed breast cancer and those who did not. Critics of the study, however, contend that all the women who took part were eating too much fat—on average, more than 30 per cent of their daily calories. They argue that if women would reduce their fat intake to under 20 per cent of their daily calories, there would be a significant decrease in the incidence of breast cancer.

Another study revealed that out of a group of women with oestrogen-sensitive tumours who have had mastectomies, those who ate a high fat diet prior to surgery were more likely to suffer a relapse of breast cancer than those who ate leaner fare.

More research is needed to determine if a very low fat diet can significantly reduce the rate of breast cancer, and at the time of writing there are some studies exploring that question. However, given the fact that a high fat diet has also been implicated in heart disease, diabetes, obesity and a host of other medical problems, I think it makes good sense to keep your daily fat intake to between 20 and 25 per cent of daily calories.

Environmental Oestrogens

For more than ten years scientists have known that certain chemicals and pollutants in the environment can disrupt normal biological processes in humans and animals. When these compounds are broken down in the body, they mimic the actions of hormones such as oestrogen and, like naturally-produced hormones, these 'chemical' hormones can trigger the growth of breast tumours and other cancers. DDT, which was once widely used as an insecticide but is now banned, is still causing trouble. DDT is broken down in the body to an even stronger compound, DDE. Studies have shown that women with breast cancer have significantly higher rates of DDE in breast tissue than women who are cancer free. DDT is not the only culprit: other compounds that can have a similar oestrogenic effect in the body include ingredients in plastics, washing detergents and some legally available pesticides.

It is very hard completely to avoid many of these chemicals because they are everywhere in our environment. However, my philosophy is that you can try to avoid as much personal contact with them as possible. For example, to reduce pesticide exposure, eat only organically grown fruits and vegetables. Organic produce is available at health food shops and some supermarkets. Although it costs a little more, I think it is worth the difference. It is also wise to avoid saturating your lawn or garden with chemicals. Fortunately there are many natural, toxin-free lawn and garden products on the market that can do the job just as well. Check with your local garden centre, health food shop or your nearest botanical gardens for information on 'environmentally friendly' gardening techniques.

Try to avoid potentially toxic household products. Although we really do not know which if any of these can increase the risk of developing breast cancer, I think it makes good sense to take some precautions. Avoid using aerosol sprays of all types— buy products that come in a spray can. Wear gloves when you are using cleaners to prevent skin contact. And avoid unnecessary products such as air fresheners.

Hormone Replacement Therapy

Millions of women take a daily dose of synthetic hormones— oestrogen and progesterone—to help alleviate some of the unpleasant symptoms and side effects of menopause. Studies show that in addition to preventing symptoms such as hot flushes, hormone replacement therapy can help prevent heart disease and osteoporosis. However, there is a downside to pumping your body full of synthetic hormones: women on hormones significantly increase their risk of breast cancer and uterine cancer—by as much as 87 per cent in the 60–66 age group. At a recent meeting of the American Association for the Advancement of Science, Dr Graham Colditz of Harvard Medical School asked an important question: 'Should breast cancer be the price we pay for reduced risk of heart disease and bone fractures?' His answer was no, and so is mine.

In the section on menopause, I described many natural and safe alternatives to hormone replacement therapy. I strongly advise women to think twice before doing anything that will increase their odds of becoming another breast cancer statistic.

Alcohol

There is a great deal of confusion about the possible link between alcohol and breast cancer. Some studies have shown that women who drink alcohol increase their odds of developing breast cancer—in a recent Spanish study of more than 760 women with breast cancer, there was evidence that even moderate drinking (one or two drinks daily) increased the risk by 50 per cent; other studies, however, have not found any connection between drinking and breast cancer.

One recent study did find a connection between alcohol intake and oestrogen levels. In a 1993 issue of the American *Journal of the National Cancer Institute*, researchers reported that women who drank about one ounce of pure alcohol daily (roughly two average drinks) showed higher blood and urine levels of oestrogen than when they abstained. Since oestrogen can promote cellular growth in breast and reproductive tissue, this is a cause for cancer, particularly among women who are already at risk. Given this information, I feel that women with family histories of breast cancer should probably drink only very occasionally, if at all. It is also advisable for women who are already taking synthetic oestrogen in the form of birth control pills or hormone replacement therapy to think twice about ingesting a substance that will boost their oestrogen levels even higher.

Fibre

Several studies have shown that a high fibre diet reduces the risk of developing breast cancer. There are several reasons why fibre may offer some protection. For one thing, foods that are high in fibre, such as fruits, vegetables and grains, tend to be low in fat. For another, these foods are also rich in phytochemicals which may help prevent the initiation and spread of many different forms of cancer. Finally, there is some evidence that a particular form of fibre, wheat bran, may help to lower the level of oestrogen. In a study conducted by the American National Health Foundation, premenopausal women were given 30 grams daily of either wheat bran, corn bran or oat bran. After two months, only the women on the wheat bran showed a significant reduction in serum oestrone and oestradiol, two potent oestrogens that are believed to stimulate the growth of breast tumours. Researchers believe that the oestrogen binds with wheat fibre and is eliminated in the faeces.

Several other foods and supplements are believed to have a protective effect against breast cancer. Below are some of these potential protectors.

Carotene. One study, performed at the Department of Social and Preventive Medicine at the State University of New York at Buffalo, compared the diets of 439 postmenopausal women with breast cancer with the diets of postmenopausal women who were cancer free. The researchers found that the risk of breast cancer was highest among women with the lowest intake of carotene in their food. Although the study appeared to deal only with beta-carotene, it is important to note that foods rich in beta-carotene are also often good sources of alpha-carotene, lutein and other carotenoids. Apricots, Chinese cabbage, pumpkin, carrots and cantaloupe are excellent sources of carotenes.

Vitamin C. Several studies have linked a low intake of vitamin C with an increased risk of breast cancer.

Genistein. Found only in soya products, this compound has been shown to block the growth of breast cancer cells in test-tube studies. Many people believe that the low rate of mortality

211

from breast cancer among Japanese women is due to their high consumption of soya products. Tofu, soya milk and soya protein are good sources of genistein.

Legumes. Legumes such as soya beans, lentils and kidney beans are also believed to protect against breast cancer. Dried beans contain many anti-cancer compounds including phytic acid and protease inhibitors. They are also low in fat.

Lignans. Found in abundance in flaxseed and to a lesser extent in rye, lignans are hormonelike compounds that compete with the body's own oestrogen for oestrogen receptor sites on cells. By doing so, lignans deactivate potent oestrogens that may trigger the growth of breast tumours.

Limonene. Found in the peel of citrus fruits, this compound has been shown to inhibit the growth of carcinogen-induced mammary tumours in rats and prevent new tumours from forming.

Omega-3 Fatty Acids. Found primarily in fatty fish such as salmon, mackerel and albacore tuna, studies have shown that omega-3 fatty acids can inhibit the growth of mammary tumours.

Quercetin. Studies show that this bioflavonoid can inhibit the growth of human tumour cells containing binding sites for Type II oestrogen, which may be responsible for some forms of breast cancer. Quercetin is abundant in red and yellow onions and shallots.

Sulphoraphane. Found in broccoli and other cruciferous vegetables, sulphoraphane promotes the production of anti-cancer enzymes in the body. In one study, rats were pretreated with either a high or a low dose of a synthetic form of sulphoraphane and then given a carcinogen known to induce mammary tumours. Another group of rats were given injections of the carcinogen only. More than two-thirds of the group which did not receive the sulphoraphane developed breast cancer, as opposed to 35 per cent of the low dose sulphoraphane treated group. Of the high dose sulphoraphane group, only 26 per cent developed cancer.

Personal Maintenance

There are no guarantees with cancer: you can do all the 'right' things, eat the right foods, take the right vitamins and, for some unknown reason, still develop breast cancer. However, the earlier the stage at which breast cancer is diagnosed, the better the prognosis. Women should be vigilant about examining their breasts for lumps or signs of abnormalities at least once a month. If you do not know how to do this, your GP or the practice nurse can show you, or you can obtain leaflets from your local well woman clinic or one of the organisations listed at the end of the book.

Many Local Health Authorities offer breast-screening to women over the age of 35. If you are offered this facility, do take it up.

Lung Cancer

FACTS Although some cases of lung cancer may be genetic or even related to diet, in many cases it is a self-inflicted disease, and cigarettes are the weapon chosen. Since women have started smoking there has been a steady rise in the incidence and mortality rate from lung cancer—in fact, since the 1980s, mortality rates from lung cancer among women have increased three per cent annually. Women smokers have more than five times the risk of developing lung cancer than non-smokers.

I know it is not easy to give up the habit. Cigarettes contain highly addictive substances that are designed to keep you coming back for more. However, bear in mind that it is not just your lungs that are in jeopardy—there is nothing that will age a woman faster than a cigarette. Women who smoke start the menopause on average two years earlier than non-smokers. They also are more prone to develop osteoporosis, acquire more wrinkles on their skin and look on average about ten years older than non-smokers.

Some forms of lung cancer are not related to smoking, and

in these cases dietary fat may be a major culprit. In a study conducted by the American National Cancer Institute, researchers surveyed 1,450 non-smokers aged 30 to 84. Out of this group, 429 had been diagnosed with lung cancer between 1986 and 1991. Based on this study, the 20 per cent of the women who ate the highest amount of saturated fat had six times the risk of developing lung cancer compared with the 20 per cent who ate the least amount. Researchers are unsure whether fat *per se* is the 'smoking gun' or whether fat was present in some other food, such as cooked red meat which also contains potential carcinogens such as heterocyclic amines.

One interesting note: in this study, the women who ate the most beans (legumes) and peas had a 40 per cent lower risk of lung cancer than those eating the least!

Saving Your Bones

FACTS Osteoporosis is caused by the thinning or wearing away of bone, which increases the susceptibility to breaks and fractures. Areas that are particularly vulnerable include vertebrae, hips and forearms. The vast majority of people with osteoporosis are women, and most of these are postmenopausal. Small-boned white and Asian women are at greatest risk of developing this disease.

Many postmenopausal women will suffer vertebral fractures and, in severe cases, some will develop a rounded back or dowager's hump, but osteoporosis is not merely an aesthetic problem: it can be very serious, even fatal. Hip fractures are a common injury among elderly women, and a number of those hospitalised for hip fractures will develop medical complications such as pneumonia or blood clots, resulting in their deaths. Osteoporosis is a growing problem already affecting one in four women. As well as fractures, it can also cause tooth loss due to bone deterioration in the jaw.

Losing bone is a natural part of the ageing process and happens in both men and women, but osteoporosis is the rapid loss of bone. During childhood and early adulthood, new bone is constantly being produced. Bone consists of several minerals including a large amount of calcium and phosphorus salts and smaller amounts of magnesium, zinc, iodine, fluoride and other trace elements. By around the age of 30, people develop their peak bone mass—that is, the production of new bone cells begins to slow down. After 35 they begin to lose roughly one per cent of their bone mass annually, but after menopause, women begin to lose about two to four per cent of their bone mass each year for up to ten years, until it starts to level off. The rapid loss after menopause is attributed to a decline in oestrogen, which is essential for calcium absorption. In fact, many menopausal women are given hormone replacement therapy (also known as oestrogen replacement therapy) because it has been shown to stem the rapid bone loss associated with menopause. However, hormone replacement therapy is a short-term solution. If a woman goes off hormones, as most do after five years, the rate of bone loss begins to accelerate. In any case, many women cannot take hormones in the first place.

Women who cannot or will not take hormones, or who do not stay on hormones for their entire postmenopausal lives, are not doomed to get osteoporosis. It is not an inevitable part of ageing and, with proper planning and intervention, can be prevented. There are many things that a woman can do throughout her lifetime to keep her bones healthy and strong.

Calcium and Vitamin D

Several studies have emphasised the need to get adequate amounts of calcium and vitamin D. The latter is essential to help the body utilise calcium and phosphorus, and some forms of osteoporosis may be caused by a genetic inability to utilise vitamin D correctly, which adversely affects the body's ability to absorb calcium. Researchers have recently isolated the gene that may be responsible for the malfunction in vitamin D.

The RDA for vitamin D is 200 iu. (Vitamin D can be toxic at levels over 1000 iu daily. Do not exceed the RDA unless under a doctor's supervision.)

The RDA for calcium is 800 mg, but some nutritionists

recommend up to 2000 mg for adults, most of whom consume roughly half the RDA. The American National Osteoporosis Foundation recommends that postmenopausal women not on hormone replacement therapy should consume 1500 mg of calcium daily. There is even some evidence that 800 mg daily may be low for girls. In one study, adolescent girls consuming about 1600 mg of calcium were shown to develop significantly stronger bone mass than girl consuming less. The researchers noted that the high calcium consumers were not excreting excess calcium in their urine, which suggested that during adolescence, when these girls were building their peak bone mass, the body was retaining the extra calcium. Although most experts do not recommend that parents give children more than 800 mg, it is imperative that children get the full RDA.

Even after peak bone mass is formed, calcium is needed to retain the bone you have. Many researchers believe that maintaining calcium levels during the 30s, 40s and 50s will help boost calcium stores which women can draw upon in later years. There is also some evidence that increasing calcium levels during menopause may make a real difference. In one 1992 French study of 3,270 women over the age of 65, researchers gave half the group supplements of 1,200 mg calcium and 800 iu of vitamin D. The other half received a placebo. After about a year and a half, the vitamin supplemented group had 43 per cent fewer hip fractures than the unsupplemented group; moreover, hip bone density had increased in the supplemented group by 2.7 per cent and had actually decreased by 4.6 per cent in the unsupplemented group.

Good food sources of calcium include low fat or fat free dairy products (one very low fat plain yogurt contains about 400 mg). However, many low fat cheeses contain phosphate which may interfere with the body's ability to absorb calcium, so these foods are not a good calcium source. Other good food sources of calcium include tofu processed with calcium sulphate (434 mg per 100 g) sardines with bones (324 mg per 75 g), calcium-fortified orange juice (22 mg per 200 ml serving) and broccoli (90 mg per 100 g, cooked). Calcium can also be obtained through supplements. There are many different types, and I recommend those that combine calcium with carbonate because they deliver a higher dose of calcium per pill than any other supplement. For maximum absorption, calcium carbonate should be taken with meals. Supplements which contain calcium citrate are also effective, but contain less calcium per dose (about 200 mg) which means that you need to take more pills. Calcium citrate should be taken on an empty stomach.

Beware of supplements made from bone meal, oyster shell or dolomite; recent studies show that they may contain unsafe levels of lead.

Vitamin D is present in fortified dairy products (one cup of milk provides 100 iu), and fatty fish oils. Sunshine is also an excellent source of vitamin D, because ultraviolet rays stimulate certain skin oils to produce vitamin D. However, sunscreens and sunblocks may filter out the rays necessary to produce vitamin D, so it is important to expose your skin to the sun without protective lotion once or twice daily, for about ten minutes. Limit this exposure to the very early morning (before 10 a.m.,) or late afternoon (after 3 p.m.,) when the sun is not at its strongest.

For many women, it may be necessary to supplement vitamin D during the winter, when bone loss occurs at a faster pace than during the warmer months. In fact, according to a recent study, a supplement of 400 iu of vitamin D during the winter can reduce bone loss. Talk to your doctor or natural healer about increasing your intake of vitamin D during the winter.

Exercise

A regular programme of weight-bearing exercise may help to strengthen bones. Indeed, the lack of physical activity in our modern lives may be one of the major reasons why osteoporosis is on the rise. Studies show that human bones are actually getting weaker. For example, during the restoration of an old church in London, scientists compared the bone density of 87 women buried in the crypt from 1729 to 1852 with the bone density of postmenopausal women living today, who were roughly the same age. The scientists discovered that the dead women had denser bones and appeared to have lost bone at a much slower rate than the present-day women. They were puzzled by the result, but attributed the denser bones of the deceased women to the fact that they were probably much more physically active than women today. Without modern conveniences such as washing machines and cars, those women performed more physically demanding tasks. Studies have shown that weight-bearing exercise, such as walking, running or jogging, can not only help build bone but will increase muscle mass, which can protect against fractures by absorbing the shock of a fall. (Swimming and cycling are not weight-bearing exercises.)

Combining calcium supplements with exercise may offer added protection. Researchers at Tufts University studied the effect of calcium and exercise on the bone density of 36 post-menopausal women. One group was given a high-calcium drink daily, containing 831 mg calcium, while the other group was given a low calcium (41 mg) placebo. Each woman was told to include 800 mg of calcium in her diet. In addition, women were either assigned to participate in an exercise group (a 50-minute walk four times per week) or were told to refrain from any recreational activity. After one year, the researchers found that the women consuming the most calcium had a two per cent increase in the femoral neck bone mineral density, whereas the placebo group had a 1.1 decrease. Not only that, the exercise group showed a 0.5 per cent increase in the bone mineral density of the spine, whereas the sedentary group experienced a seven per cent decline. This and other similar studies show that diet and lifestyle can make a significant difference in reducing the risk of osteoporosis.

Other Bone Builders

There are other foods and supplements that may help to preserve bone, including:

Boron. Researchers at USDA found that a supplement of 3 mg of boron daily could double serum oestrogen levels in women, which might help to prevent osteoporosis. Oestrogen helps to retain adequate amounts of calcium and magnesium which are needed to build strong bones. Good food sources of boron include dried fruit and grapes.

Soya Foods. Even though Japanese women are small-boned, they suffer about half the number of hip injuries of Western women. The fact that they have more physical activity may be one reason why they have fewer injuries. For example, Japanese women typically sit on the floor, and the action of getting up and down several times daily may help to develop their hip bones. However, their diet, which is rich in soya foods, may be another reason why they have stronger bones. Researchers at the University of North Carolina investigated the effect of genistein, which is found in soya beans, on the bone mass of rats who had their ovaries removed to eliminate their natural source of oestrogen. Genistein is rich in plant oestrogens, compounds which mimic the action of natural oestrogen in the body. The study determined that genistein was able to prevent bone loss in rats almost as well as a synthetic form of oestrogen. Although more studies need to be done, soya appears to be a bone-sparing food that all women should include in their diet. (Tofu made with calcium sulphate is a particularly good choice: it is abundant in both calcium and genistein.)

Watch These Bone Breakers

Caffeine can hamper calcium absorption. In a four-year study performed at the University of California with nearly 1,000 postmenopausal women, researchers found that those who drank two cups of coffee per day or more suffered a significant drop in bone density. However, those who drank at least one cup of milk per day seemed to be protected from coffee's bone-breaking effect.

Smokers have a higher rate of osteoporosis than non-smokers. Yet another reason to kick the habit!

Alcohol can hamper the absorption of calcium, which will cause bones to become thin and brittle. Excessive drinking also makes you more prone to falling, which can result in a break or fracture.

Chapter 5

Just for Men

Men typically die younger than women. I don't believe that men are the 'weaker sex', rather that they are more stoic about their health—they often ignore important symptoms and deal with health problems only when they absolutely have to (or when their wives force them to!). However, a new generation of men is taking a greater interest in health and fitness, and I believe this change in attitude may add years to the average man's life span. Here is some important information that every man should know.

Sexual Health

FACTS Good health and great sex go hand in hand at any age, but it is particularly true for men once they reach middle age. As men approach the second half of life, hormonal shifts and other changes can alter sexual response. Hormone levels that control sexual arousal may dip. For example, many men show a marked drop in testosterone production beginning around their late forties—this period is called viropause and there are some similarities to the female menopause. In the same way, some men may experience minor symptoms resulting from hormonal fluctuations. Although men remain fertile, they may find that it takes longer to get an erection and they may have difficulty maintaining one at times. However, none of these factors should significantly impair a man's ability to enjoy sex.

There is no intrinsic reason why a man cannot enjoy a vigorous sex life throughout his entire life, but many men do not. According to the Massachusetts Male Ageing Study, a recent groundbreaking study of men between the ages of 40 and 70, about half of the 1,290 participants experienced some form of impotency. The researchers defined impotency as 'the persistent inability to attain and maintain an erection adequate to permit satisfactory sexual performance'. Most of the men experienced minimal or moderate forms of impotency and the risk of severe or total impotency increased threefold with age: 5.1 per cent of all 40-year-olds complained of complete impotency, as against 15 per cent of all 70-year-olds. But the researchers were quick to point out that in most cases, a persistent sexual problem was a sign of an underlying physical problem. In fact, 39 per cent of the heart disease patients and 15 per cent of the patients diagnosed with high blood pressure were completely impotent, compared with less than ten per cent of the entire group. (In these situations, the impotency is often not due to the disease, but to the medication that is used to treat it, as I shall discuss later.) Disregard for one's body also seemed to be a major culprit in promoting impotency. For example, for heart patients, smoking appeared to be the kiss of death for sex: those who smoked were three times more likely to be impotent than those who did not.

The study also revealed that the men least likely to complain of impotency were those with high levels of HDLs or 'good' cholesterol, and that, contrary to popular opinion, blood testosterone levels were not related to male potency. But another hormone was right on target: blood levels of dehydroepiandrosterone (DHEA), which is produced by the pituitary, were a good indicator of impotency (for more information on DHEA, see p. 146). In fact, men with the highest levels of DHEA were the least likely to be impotent. This does not mean that DHEA promotes sexuality; its effect on a man's sex life may simply be due to the fact that men with high DHEA levels are less likely to develop heart disease.

Many of the physical problems that can destroy a man's sex life are easily avoidable, or can be successfully treated. Here are some of the major causes of male impotency, and ways of coping with them.

221

POOR CIRCULATION

In order to maintain an erection, blood must flow freely to the penis. However, if the arteries delivering blood to the genitals become narrowed or clogged due to atherosclerosis, the blood supply will be impaired. This could explain why so many heart patients complain of impotency. Diabetics, hypertensives and heavy smokers are also at great risk of damage to their vascular system, which could result in a poor blood flow to their genitals. Impotency is often the first sign of a circulatory problem in men.

Recommendations

A low fat diet (with less than 20 per cent of your daily calories in the form of fat) is your best defence against 'clogged arteries'. If you smoke, stop. Each and every cigarette you smoke inflicts slow damage on your vascular system which will eventually result in circulatory problems. In addition, if you smoke, your partner may well do, too. Smoking can impair a woman's vaginal lubrication, which will make having sex even more difficult.

If you are diabetic, be especially vigilant about maintaining normal blood sugar levels—there is evidence that high blood sugar can cause nerve damage which may contribute to impotency. The combination of cigarette smoking and diabetes appears to be particularly dangerous.

To improve blood flow throughout the body, including the sex organs, take a vitamin E supplement of 400 iu twice daily, morning and evening. (Do not take vitamin E if you are taking a blood thinner.) The Chinese herb *Ginkgo biloba* has also been shown to improve circulation to the extremities. *Ginkgo biloba* is available in capsule form at health food shops.

ALCOHOL

Although a drink or two may help you 'loosen up', contrary to popular belief alcohol actually inhibits erection and ejaculation in men. Heavy drinkers may damage their liver, thus impairing the production of sex hormones, and chronic alcoholics may permanently damage nerves within their penis which are essential to maintain an erection.

Recommendations

If sex is on your agenda, keep the alcohol for afterwards. If you are a heavy drinker, talk to your doctor about getting help to stop.

DRUGS

Prescription and over-the-counter drugs can cause many sexual problems in men. Some medications, including those used to treat high blood pressure, depression, anxiety and even allergies, can sap sexual desire or cause impotency or difficulty with ejaculation. For example, some men on beta blockers (used to treat hypertension) may experience what I call the beta blocker blues, a palpable loss in libido; and men on antidepressant drugs may suffer a loss of libido and find that they have difficulty with ejaculation. Some men may respond to certain medications with excessive fatigue—although they may be physically capable of having sex, they may feel too exhausted.

Recommendations

I don't want to alarm men who may be on prescription drugs: these kinds of adverse reactions are relatively rare, affecting between one and two per cent of users. However, if a man is experiencing impotency or other sexual problems and is taking medication, he should consult his doctor to determine whether the medication could be causing the problem. Often, simply switching to another medication will solve the problem. **If you are on medication for heart disease, high blood pressure or any other serious problem, do not discontinue your medication without first consulting your doctor.**

If you are hypertensive and suspect that your blood pressure medication is bringing you down, it may be possible to reduce your dose simply by making certain changes in your diet and lifestyle (see p. 181). Be sure to work closely with your doctor or natural healer so that he or she can monitor your results.

If you are taking medication for a heart problem, bear in mind that fear may be hampering your sexual performance, not your medication. Many heart patients mistakenly believe that they cannot withstand the physical stress of sex. In most cases this is simply not true. In fact, one recent study concluded that for most heart patients, having sex was no more dangerous than getting out of bed in the morning! Talk to your doctor or natural healer about your fears.

FATIGUE, LOSS OF DESIRE

If you simply can't summon up the energy (or the interest) to have sex, you need to re-examine your lifestyle. Are you getting enough sleep? Are you getting enough exercise? Are you eating a healthy diet? Are you knocking yourself out at night with a nightcap? Could you be suffering from a vitamin deficiency? Excessive fatigue could be a sign of depression or an underlying physical problem, so if you are constantly exhausted, you should consult your doctor or natural healer. However, very often it is a sign of poor nutrition and poor health habits.

Recommendations

Be sure you are getting enough of the following:

Vitamin A. Vitamin A helps produce sex hormones that are essential for sexual functioning. Eat foods rich in beta-carotene, which is converted into vitamin A as the body needs it. Take 10,000 to 15,000 iu of beta-carotene daily.

Vitamin B$_6$. This vitamin increases the hormone that regulates testosterone. Good food sources include brewer's yeast, wheat germ, cantaloupe, cabbage and blackstrap molasses. A good multivitamin will contain B$_6$.

Manganese. This mineral helps to produce two chemicals in the brain that heighten sexual arousal—dopamine and acetyl-choline. Good food sources of manganese include nuts, whole grain breads, cereals, legumes, beets and green leafy vegetables.

Zinc. Zinc is essential for the production of testosterone. (As I shall discuss later, it also helps to keep the prostate gland healthy.) Men should take between 15–50 mg of zinc daily.

Octacosanol. This natural food supplement, which is rich in wheat, wheat germ and vegetable oils, is reputed to increase stamina and sexual performance in some men. Octacosanol is sold in capsule form in health food shops.

Yohimbe. This herb is the only officially approved aphrodisiac on the market for men. The drug yohimbine is available only on prescription and has been shown to restore sexual potency in some men. The herb yohimbe, a much weaker version of the drug, is available in health food shops and is included in many so-called 'male potency' formulae. I recommend 500 mg capsules, up to two or three times daily.

Following my simple suggestions may help some men. However, any man who has a chronic problem with impotency should see his doctor or natural healer. Fortunately there are numerous medical treatments available for impotency, including surgical penile implants. Don't suffer in silence, talk to your doctor.

Prostate Problems

FACTS The prostate is a small, walnut-sized gland located between the bladder and the penis above the rectum. The prostate gland produces semen, the fluid that carries sperm. During childhood, the prostate is tiny, but once puberty starts and testosterone levels rise, the prostate gland grows to adult size. The gland remains stable until around the age of 45, at which time it often experiences a second growth spurt. By the age of 60, most men have an enlarged prostate gland, a condition which is called benign prostate hypertrophy (BPH). As its name implies, in most cases BPH is harmless although it can be quite annoying. If the prostate gland becomes very swollen, it can push against the urethra and interfere with urination. In fact, in about ten per cent of all men, the first sign of BPH is urinary retention. Other symptoms include difficulty or straining during urination and frequent urination, especially at night. In severe cases, urine can gather in the bladder until it eventually backs up into the kidneys, causing kidney damage. About ten per cent of men with BPH will require corrective surgery—in fact, prostate surgery is the most common surgery performed on people over 64.

Some men may find that certain foods, such as caffeinated beverages, alcoholic drinks and hot, spicy food may aggravate their condition. Obviously, if you find certain foods or drinks irritating, your best bet is to avoid them. However, many men with BPH try to cope with their problem by drastically reducing their intake of liquids. This is not a good idea, and could actually add to their woes by triggering a urinary tract infection. If you have BPH, consult with your doctor or natural healer. Most men can be treated successfully with medication, or with any number of interesting herbal remedies that may relieve some of their discomfort.

Recommendations

Health food shops are filled with prostate remedies, some of which work well for many men. Natural remedies tend to work better in the early stages of BPH. The advantage of using natural remedies is that they are inexpensive and can be purchased without a prescription; the downside is that they are much weaker than the prescription drugs and may not work for everybody. On the positive side, however, they do not cause any known side effects. For many men, herbal remedies will do the trick. However, if the herbal remedy does not help, they can always switch to a stronger medication. The following is a list of some popular herbal remedies that may help men with BPH.

Saw Palmetto. Many herbal formulae for BPH contain extract from the berries of the saw palmetto tree. Native Americans ate saw palmetto berries as part of their diet, and natural healers have long prescribed these berries for urinary problems.

Several studies have shown that saw palmetto can increase the flow of urine and reduce night-time urination in men with BPH. In Europe, where most of the research on saw palmetto has been conducted, this herb is an accepted treatment for BPH.

Some studies show that saw palmetto berry extract may work by preventing the conversion of testosterone to its more potent form, dihydrotestosterone. Compounds in the saw palmetto berry may block dihydrotestosterone's ability to bind to receptor sites on prostate cells, thus preventing the cells from growing. Take one to three capsules (540 mg) daily.

Pygeum. The bark of the pygeum plant has been used for prostate problems since the eighteenth century and is included in many modern herbal formulae. Pygeum contains phytosterols, compounds that have anti-inflammatory activity. Phytosterols block the production of prostaglandins, compounds involved in the inflammatory process. In addition, pygeum is a diuretic which can help promote urination.

Pumpkin or Squash Seed. A species of pumpkin or squash grown in the Near East (*Cucurbita pepo*) is included in many herbal prostate formulae. *Cucurbita pepo* contain many beneficial phytochemicals including betasistosterol, an anti-inflammatory, and cucurbitacin, which may help facilitate urination by relaxing the sphincter (which regulates the flow of urine) and increasing the tone of bladder muscles. Pumpkin seeds are also an excellent source of vitamin E and zinc.

Pumpkin seed oil is also sold in health food shops in capsule form.

Stinging Nettle. This herb is a diuretic and anti-inflammatory. It is often used in conjunction with the herbs discussed above to treat prostate problems.

Couch Grass. This mild diuretic is often included in herbal combinations for BPH.

The Role of Zinc. Zinc plays a major role in the male reproductive system and there are heavy concentrations in the prostate gland. Zinc stimulates the production of testosterone, the male hormone which aids in the function of erection and ejaculation. A zinc deficiency may contribute to infertility. Zinc may also help to prevent BPH. I therefore advise men to take 15–50 mg of zinc daily and to eat foods rich in zinc, which include pumpkin seeds, oysters, cashews, non-fat dry milk, brown mustard, loin of pork, lean steak and brewer's yeast.

CANCER OF THE PROSTATE

Cancer of the prostate is a common form of male cancer, and in most cases, if caught early, it can be successfully treated by surgery or radiation therapy. In many older men (over 60), however, the tumours are so slow growing that they may not need treatment at all. In these cases the doctor may recommend a policy of 'watchful waiting' to see how the cancer progresses.

Because of the risk of prostate cancer, men over 40 should have an annual physical examination which includes a digital rectal exam. In this exam, the physician inserts a lubricated finger into the rectum to palpate for any prostate irregularities or early rectal cancers. However, the digital rectal exam may not detect small tumours and it is a good idea for men over 50 also to have an annual prostate specific antigen blood test. Prostate specific antigen is a protein produced by the prostate, and high levels may be a sign of tumour growth.

All men should be aware of the following warning signs and symptoms of prostate cancer and should report them to their doctors:

- Any changes in urinary habits.
- The presence of blood in the urine.
- Painful urination.
- Continuing pain in the lower back, pelvis or upper thighs.

Keep in mind that having one or more of these symptoms does not mean that you have cancer. It could also be a sign of a urinary tract infection or another problem and should not be ignored. Even if it does turn out to be prostate cancer, the earlier the diagnosis, the better the prognosis.

In the United States and Britain, prostate cancer is relatively common, but not so in Asia or Africa. Indeed, Japanese men have the lowest rate of mortality from prostate cancer in the world. Native Nigerians have a lower rate of prostate cancer than African American men in the United States. Researchers suspect that diet and other environmental factors may contribute to the risk of dying from prostate cancer.

In one major study of 48,000 men, conducted at Harvard Medical School, researchers found that diet may play a major role in determining who lives or dies from prostate cancer. In this study, researchers compared the diets of the 417 men out of the group who had been diagnosed with prostate cancer with the eating habits of those who did not get this disease. They found that diet did not appear to increase the odds of developing prostate cancer, but among the men who developed this disease, a diet high in fat seemed to be a major factor in dictating whether or not the disease progressed to a more advanced state. Animal fat in particular appeared to have a lethal effect on prostate cancer—men who ate the highest amounts of red meat, butter and chicken with skin fared the worst. However, eating skinless chicken, vegetable fat or dairy products other than butter seemed to have no adverse affect. From this information, researchers concluded that a particular form of fatty acid—alpha linolenic acid found in animal sources—may be responsible for triggering tumour growth. It is interesting to note that other studies have shown that Seventh Day Adventist men, who follow a vegetarian diet, have a much lower rate of prostate cancer than the national average. And even though Japanese men have an extremely low rate of mortality from prostate cancer while living in Japan, when they migrate to the United States—and presumably begin eating the typical American diet—their risk dramatically increases

Another reason why Japanese men in Japan may be protected against prostate cancer is the fact that their diet is rich in soys foods such as tofu and soya milk. Numerous studies have shown that many of the compounds in soya have potent anti-cancer properties. Soya is rich in phyto-oestrogens, hormonelike compounds that may deactivate the more potent hormones that can trigger tumour growth. One compound in particular, genistein, has been shown in test-tube studies to inhibit the growth of prostate tumour cells. Genistein is now being tested on men in the United States, who are in the early stages of prostate cancer, to see if it can slow down the progress of the disease. Interestingly enough, autopsies of Japanese men reveal that their rate of prostate cancer is as high as that of American men—most of them have small tumours in their prostates when they die—but the tumours are not detected because they are so slow-growing, they never develop into clinical disease. Studies will show whether or not genistein is the 'secret weapon' against prostate cancer, but meanwhile I recommend that men try to eat at least one serving (50–75g) of tofu or soya food daily. I start my morning with a tofu shake. There are also powdered soya protein products on the market that offer a day's supply of genistein. (For more information see p. 65.)

Other Male Concerns

HAIR TODAY...

Some men manage to keep a thick head of hair throughout their entire lives, but most men starting around middle age or even younger, experience hair loss which may eventually lead to balding. Young, healthy men lose an average of about 100 hairs daily, which are usually replaced by new growth. As men age, however, hair may tend to thin out and, in some cases, result in balding.

About two-thirds of all men have male pattern baldness, which is a genetic condition passed down by either parent. However, even if one of your parents is bald, it does not mean that your fate is sealed: the gene can skip a generation. On the other hand, the reverse is also true: even if your parents have thick, lustrous manes you could still inherit the gene for baldness.

Male pattern baldness usually begins gradually, starting with a loss of hair on the front of the scalp at either side of the hairline or on the crown, the circular area on top. Hair loss can start as early as the teenage years, but more often than not it begins during middle age.

Why so many otherwise healthy men lose their hair as they age is still very much a mystery. Some researchers believe that testosterone, the male hormone, may thwart hair growth by shrinking the hair follicle. Others believe that the hair follicle becomes clogged with sebum, a substance produced by the skin, which prevents nutrients from reaching the hair follicle, thus thwarting growth.

In some cases, hair loss may be caused by an underlying physical problem. For example, an underactive or an overactive thyroid can create a hormonal imbalance that may accelerate hair loss, but once the problem is corrected the hair grows back. Cancer patients may suffer temporary hair loss after radiation or chemotherapy treatments. Sometimes rapid hair loss is a sign of an autoimmune disease called alopecia areata, which results in patchy bald spots on the scalp. However, hair loss due to alopecia is usually temporary in adults. In extremely rare cases a severe vitamin deficiency may be the underlying cause.

For thousands of years men have sought a cure for baldness, but even today there is no tried and true cure for this problem. However, there are some treatments that may help some people.

Jojoba Oil (pronounced Ho-ho-ba), which is made from a desert plant, can improve the blood flow to the scalp. After shampooing, massage a few drops of oil into your scalp and keep on overnight. Be sure to avoid contact with your eyes, and if any irritation occurs, discontinue use. Shampoo out in the morning.

Diet and Nutrition play a major role in how you feel, and how you feel is reflected in how you look. Although a healthy lifestyle may not prevent hair loss, it can help keep your remaining hair in peak condition. For a healthy, shining mane, be sure to eat foods rich in B vitamins. Brewer's yeast, wheat germ oil, raw or roasted nuts or whole grain foods are packed with B vitamins.

As the baby boom generation grows up—the generation that turned long hair into a political statement—there is likely to be a frantic search for a cure for baldness. One Canadian company is even experimenting with a machine that zaps the scalp with low-level electricity which supposedly stems hair loss by stimulating the hair follicles.

When it comes to balding, men will try practically anything. The Native Americans used to rub chilli peppers on their scalp to stimulate hair growth. This is not as crazy as it sounds: chilli peppers stimulate blood flow to the hair follicles, allowing nutrients to flow freely. I don't recommend this treatment because chilli peppers can be very irritating to the skin and eyes, but it is interesting to note that the so-called hot new treatments of today are not really that 'hot' or 'new'.

SAVE YOUR SKIN

Skin cancer, in its potentially lethal form of melanoma, afflicts men more than women. Not so coincidentally, men spend nearly twice as much time in the sun as do women and are four times less likely to use a sunscreen.

I can't stress this enough—if you are exposed to the sun, you must use a sunscreen of at least 15 SPF at all times. Make sure that the sunscreen offers broad spectrum protection, which means that it filters out both UVA and UVB rays.

Remember that sunscreens are not a panacea. Recent studies show that although sunscreens can help prevent basal cell and squamous skin cancers, both of which are highly treatable if caught early, they do not protect against the more serious melanoma. Try to avoid sun exposure during the 'burning rays' of 11 a.m. to 2 p.m. However, if you spend a great deal of time outdoors, for example, if you work outside during the summer months, I recommend wearing sun-protective clothing. Dark clothing with a heavy weave offers the best protection, although it is likely that it will also keep you uncomfortably warm. A summer weight T-shirt offers protection equal to an SPA of 5–7, and only an SPA 2 when it is wet. Fortunately, there are some new lines of lightweight clothes that are specifically designed to offer additional sun protection. There are at least three manufacturers that claim their outerwear offers an SPF of 30. Look for sun-protective clothing at your local sports goods supplier.

Don't forget to wear a hat—it not only offers additional protection for your face, but shields your scalp from the cancer-causing rays.

Men who feel that summer is not summer without a tan should consider using a self-tanning cream. In the past these creams fell into disrepute because they turned the skin a sallow, yellow colour. However, the new creams produce a better result and in my opinion are a much safer alternative to a suntan.

SAVE YOUR BLADDER

It is conventional wisdom that people should drink between eight and ten glasses of water daily, and I know many active men who drink even more. Water helps prevent constipation, keeps the skin moist and helps maintain the correct balance of fluids in the body. A recent study, however, showed that men who drink 14 or more cups of fluid daily of any kind—including coffee or fruit juice—face two to four times greater risk of developing bladder cancer than men who drink around seven cups. Further investigation showed that tap water—whether consumed in pure form, or diluted in fruit juice or brewed coffee—appeared to be the culprit. Researchers suggest that chlorine in municipal water systems may promote cancer. My advice: go on drinking water, especially in the hot, summer months, but switch to bottled water, or install a home filtering system (see Water, p. 138).

Testosterone

At one time, researchers believed that the male hormone testosterone was the main reason why men fell prey to heart disease at younger ages and had a shorter life span than women. However, recent studies suggest that testosterone may have been getting a bad press. For example, one important study performed at

St Luke's-Roosevelt Hospital Center in New York showed that, contrary to previous assumptions, men with lower levels of testosterone were more likely to get heart disease than men with higher levels. Moreover, men with higher testosterone levels had higher levels of HDL or 'good' cholesterol.

Testosterone levels tend to decline with age, and some researchers speculate that providing supplemental testosterone to men with low levels may help to ward off some age-related ailments. For example, studies have shown that testosterone supplements in older men may help to prevent osteoporosis, maintain muscle strength, control depression, increase sex drive and even help to boost brain function. Some researchers speculate that in the not too distant future, many older men may routinely take testosterone supplements in much the same way that menopausal women take oestrogen replacement therapy. There is one downside to testosterone: like oestrogen, it can stimulate the growth of hormone-sensitive tumours and may contribute to prostate cancer. My advice: good as testosterone therapy may sound, proceed with caution.

Chapter 6

The Power of Exercise

Since early times men and women have been desperately search-ing for a fountain of youth—a magical pill or potion that could reverse the ageing process. Fortunately the search is over and the fountain of youth may be as close as your local gym.

Study after study confirms that exercise may be the only true way to turn back the clock. I am not talking about becoming a marathon runner or an Olympic athlete; a moderate and consist-ent exercise programme is all it takes to live longer, live stronger and live better.

As we age there are many physical changes that affect our strength and appearance. For most people, by the age of 45, there is a noticeable decline in muscle mass and an increase in body fat—in fact the typical sedentary adult loses up to three kilos of lean body mass every ten years. There is also a decrease in bone density; bones get thinner and more prone to fracture. Aerobic ability declines, which means that you may find yourself huffing and puffing more after exertion. There is also a loss of flexibility—you may feel stiffer and less supple. However, age-ing does not have to be a physical downward spiral. Many of these changes can be postponed, minimised and even reversed by physical activity. Experts say that a fit fifty- or sixty-year-old can actually be in better shape than a flabby thirty-year-old! Exercise may also help to prevent many of the diseases that can cut life short.

Longevity

A recent study of 10,000 Harvard graduates aged 45–84 showed that those who participated in moderately vigorous activities (such as tennis, swimming, jogging or brisk walking) had up to a 29 per cent lower death rate than the sedentary men. On average, exercisers lived ten months longer than those who did not exercise, and even those who began exercising late in life (after the age of 65) lived up to six months longer than couch potatoes.

In another study performed at the Institute for Aerobics Research and the Cooper Clinic in Dallas, researchers followed 13,000 men and women for an average of eight years to determine whether there was any correlation between fitness levels and longevity. Based on the results of an exercise treadmill test, the group was divided into five levels ranging from the least fit to the most fit. The women in the least fit group had the highest mortality rate, but the women in the second lowest fitness group had nearly half the death rate of the least fit. Based on these findings, the researchers concluded that something as easy as taking a brisk walk every day could add years to your life.

Heart

In the Harvard study of 10,000 men, those who exercised had a 41 per cent reduced risk of heart disease compared with sedentary men. This is not surprising since other studies have shown that regular exercise can decrease your total cholesterol, increase the 'good' HDLs, improve respiratory function and lower your blood pressure. In another study conducted at the Laboratory of Cardiovascular Science at the Gerontology Research Center, Baltimore, researchers found that physical activity may retard the increased stiffness in arteries that often accompanies ageing. The scientists studied 14 middle-aged long distance runners who ran about ten miles a week. They found that the runners had a greater capacity to dilate their coronary arteries than sedentary men of the same age, thus markedly increasing the blood flow to their hearts. Researchers are not sure how much activity is required to keep arteries from stiffening, but they do know that being sedentary is a sure way to speed up the process.

Stroke

In a 22-year follow-up of more than 5,300 Japanese Americans in the famous Honolulu Heart study, researchers found a strong association between a sedentary lifestyle and an increased risk of stroke. The study suggested that exercise may protect non-smokers against stroke. In active and partially inactive men between the ages of 55 and 68, there was a four-fold risk of haemorrhagic stroke (bleeding in the brain) and a three-fold risk of subarachnoid stroke (bleeding between the brain and the skull) compared to active men.

Exercise also appears to protect women against stroke. Researchers at the University of Washington in Seattle investigated exercise intensity and early signs of cardiovascular disease in about 1,200 women. The scientists found that the women who exercised the least were most likely to show signs of thickening of the inner and middle layers of the carotid arteries in the neck, which could increase the risk of stroke.

Cancer

Exercise appears to offer a protective effect against different forms of cancer. Many animal studies have shown that exercise can inhibit tumour growth and there is some evidence that increased physical activity may harm cancer cells. For example, a recent study showed that men with sedentary jobs were 1.6 times more likely to develop colon cancer than those with more active jobs. Researchers speculate that physical activity causes an increased motility of the gastrointestinal tract and more frequent bowel movements, which limits exposure to potential carcinogens in stool.

There is also a link between exercise and lower rates of breast cancer. In a major study performed at Harvard School of Public Health, researchers tracked the exercise habits of 5,400 women graduates aged 21–80. According to this study, the more athletic the woman, the lower her risk of developing breast cancer. Other studies have shown that exercise can reduce oestrogen levels—some forms of oestrogen can trigger the growth of tumour cells.

Immunity

Exercise may add some zest to your immune system. Exercise heats up the body, in much the same way that a fever raises your temperature. When the body is warm it triggers the production of pyrogen, a protein which is part of the interleukins, the white blood cells that enhance immune function. Other studies suggest that exercise may reverse the drop in immune function that normally occurs with ageing. Researchers at Appalachian State University found that very fit women over 70 had immune systems that functioned as well as women half their age!

A word of caution: long distance running may actually dampen your immune system. Studies show that runners are more prone to colds, flu and upper respiratory ailments after participating in a marathon. Researchers suspect that overexertion may have a weakening effect on the body. Moderation is the key!

Preventing Frailty

Researchers are learning that exercise can keep you active and mobile at any age. According to a groundbreaking study conducted at the Hebrew Rehabilitation Programme for the Aged in Boston, a carefully planned strength-training programme for the elderly can counteract the muscle weakness typical of very old people. The study found an average 113 per cent increase in muscle strength among the participants, which in many cases meant the difference between eating alone in their rooms or being able to walk to the dining-room. On average, the exercisers experienced a 12 per cent increase in walking speed and a 28 per cent increase in stair-climbing power. An added bonus: the people who exercised began to take part in more recreational and educational activities offered at the home, thus enriching their lives in other ways. Researchers suspect that if more older people participated in strength-training programmes, many could avoid the falls and injuries that force them into nursing homes in the first place. Other studies have shown that men as old as 90-plus showed a significant improvement in muscle strength after a mere eight weeks of exercise.

Mental Fitness

Flexing your muscles may strengthen your brain power. Researchers have documented that older people who do regular aerobic exercise perform significantly better in cognitive tests than their sedentary colleagues. One explanation could be that exercise improves the flow of blood to the brain.

Mental Well-being

Exercise makes you happier. Physical activity increases the release of beta-endorphins, chemicals produced by the brain that are natural pain-killers. Exercise also lowers your adrenaline level, which can reduce feelings of stress and anxiety.

Building Bone

Weightbearing exercise can help slow down the loss of bone mass which is particularly problematic in postmenopausal women. Researchers suspect that regular exercise could help women retain up to five per cent of their bone mass—women on average lose up to 35 per cent of their bone mass in the years following menopause. Beginning an exercise programme before menopause will lay down a foundation of bigger and stronger bones.

GETTING STARTED

Take Thirty

Fifty per cent of the population are sedentary—that is, they barely get any physical activity at all. Many people say that they would like to exercise, but with their busy schedules they simply cannot find time during the day to work out. Many were also put off by exercise gurus who insisted that fitness could only be achieved by following a complicated and rigorous programme. The good news is that they were wrong: all it takes to achieve a reasonable level of fitness is to exercise moderately for at least 30 minutes more or less every day. It does not have to be in one continuous session—you can do a little bit of exercise throughout the day so long as it adds up to a total of 30 minutes.

Design an exercise programme that works best for you. For example, it can be as simple as taking a brisk fifteen-minute walk twice daily (or three walks of ten minutes apiece). Or you can work out on an exercise bike for fifteen minutes in the morning before work, and take a fifteen-minute walk after work. Have a back-up plan for bad weather. An indoor jogging track or shopping mall is a great place to walk or run on wet days. Don't worry if you miss a day—so long as you exercise on most days you are ahead of the game. Jogging, running, tennis and swimming are also good choices. Or try something more exotic, such as fencing or martial arts. Many older people are discovering that studying T'ai Chi can help build strength, grace, endurance and confidence.

Stretching

In addition to the thirty-minute activity programme, I recommend that everyone should do some simple stretching exercises at least three times a week for fifteen minutes at a time, to help maintain flexibility. It is not difficult: simply get down on the floor and gently stretch and flex every joint and bone in your body. Start with your toes and work your way up. Breathe slowly and deeply into the stretch, and stop if you feel any pain or discomfort. Even better, join a stretch and tone class at a local health club. Even if you attend just one stretch class weekly, you can still do the exercises at home on your own. There are also some excellent exercise videos on the market, which include stretching and strengthening.

Strength Training

Several studies have shown that strength training with weights can preserve flexibility, muscle and bone in people well into their nineties. I do not recommend buying a set of weights and working out on your own—the chance of injury is too great—but I do recommend learning how to use weights properly at a health club. Hire a personal trainer to work with you for a few sessions so that you can learn how to use weights safely. In some cases the club may even provide new members with a few free sessions with a trainer. Check up on the club's credentials before you join.

Helpful Tips

Find an exercise partner. It is more fun to have company, and you are less likely to slack off if another person is counting on you. It is also safer to run or walk with someone else, but even with a partner avoid walking in deserted areas. Be sure to wear reflective gear at night, especially if you are walking on a road used by cars.

If you have a heart condition or any other medical problem, consult your doctor before beginning an exercise programme.

ARE YOU GETTING ENOUGH OF WHAT YOU NEED?

Exercise places new demands on your body. Be sure that you are getting enough of these important vitamins and minerals.

Chromium Picolinate. Chromium helps to burn fat and regulate blood sugar. Combined with exercise, it can help build muscle. Many people are deficient in chromium. Good food sources include spices such as cinnamon, grape juice, brewer's yeast, broccoli, mushrooms, whole wheat, apples and peanuts. Chromium picolinate supplements are sold in health food shops. Take 200 mcg capsules or tablets up to three times daily.

B_2 (Riboflavin). This B vitamin helps the body release energy from food. Researchers at Cornell University found that the

need for riboflavin increases with activity. Many studies show that older people do not get enough of this vitamin. Good food sources include low fat milk, yogurt, lean beef, fortified breads and cereals and green vegetables. Riboflavin is included in many multivitamins and B supplements. Take 50–100 mg daily.

Vitamin E. Although exercise offers many benefits, several studies have shown that vigorous exercise increases oxygen consumption, which may promote the formation of free radicals, unstable molecules that can destroy cells. However, antioxidants, particularly vitamin E, may help prevent this damage, and studies also show that vitamin E supplements can help prevent muscle soreness that often occurs after a work-out. It is difficult to get enough vitamin E from food alone, so I recommend taking 800 iu daily in the form of D-alpha tocopheryl succinate (dry form.)

Potassium. Sweating can sap the body of important minerals, including sodium, of which most of us have enough and to spare, and potassium which can be replaced by eating potassium-rich foods. Fruits such as bananas, orange juice and prunes are excellent sources of potassium. So are baked white potatoes and plain yogurt.

Water. While you are exercising, take a few sips of water every ten minutes or so. Do not forget to drink at least two glasses of water after working out.

Zinc. Increased physical activity can lead to a loss of zinc in sweat and urine. Zinc-rich foods include pumpkin seeds, oysters, low fat milk, brewer's yeast and lamb chops. Zinc is included in many multivitamins. Take 15–50 mg daily.

Chapter 7

Looking Good and Staying that Way

Nothing can make you look older than wrinkled, dried-out skin. But skin is not just for decoration: it is actually the largest organ system in the body and one of the most hard-working. Skin performs many critical tasks: it helps regulate body temperature, it enables the body to retain fluids and it is the immune system's first line of defence against viruses, bacteria and other foreign objects.

As we age, skin undergoes normal wear and tear. Fine lines and wrinkles may develop, caused primarily by a breakdown in collagen, the protein responsible for the support and elasticity of the skin. Gravity begins to pull the skin down, which can cause it to loosen and become flabby. The body produces less sebum, an oil that forms a protective coating around the skin, which can result in patches of dry, itchy skin. Cell regeneration slows down, leaving the skin looking drab and tired. Perhaps the worst assault of all on skin is caused by exposure to ultraviolet light from sunlight, which can damage skin cells and cause signs of premature ageing and skin cancer.

Until recently we believed that little could be done to prevent the skin from showing signs of age. We now know, however, that a combination of factors, including lifestyle, diet, supplements and skin care products can help skin maintain a youthful appearance and, more importantly, keep it cancer free.

GETTING BACK TO BASICS

Healthy habits are reflected in healthy, glowing skin. Before investing a lot of money in fancy products, try these simple tips.

Beauty is From the Inside Out

Skin is made of cells, and cells need the proper nutrients to thrive. A careful diet including an abundance of fruits, vegetables and fibre can help keep your body working well and your skin in top form. Studies have also shown that a low fat diet (no more than 20 per cent of your calories from fat) can reduce the risk of developing precancerous skin lesions (actinic keratoses) that can lead to non-melanoma skin cancer. Vitamins and other supplements can also help. In particular, I recommend:

> RECIPE FOR BEAUTIFUL SKIN
> SOD (superoxide dismutase) and Wild Yams—300 mg each daily
> Cysteine—500 mg
> Vitamin C—1500 mg
> Biotin—100 mcg
> Beta-carotene—25,000 iu
> Water—six–eight glasses daily of filtered or bottled water

Get Your Beauty Sleep

During sleep our bodies secrete human growth hormone and other skin growth factors which may stimulate the production of collagen and the production of new skin cells. A chronic lack of sleep may take its toll on your complexion.

Smoking

According to a report in the *New England Journal of Medicine*, smokers are more likely to appear at least five years older than non-smokers. Smoking is associated with an acceleration in facial wrinkling, perhaps because smokers are constantly squinting their eyes to avoid smoke from their own cigarettes.

Water

If you don't get enough fluids, your body will sap fluid out of body cells, which can leave them dehydrated. Dehydrated skin cells are more likely to have a dried-up, wrinkled appearance. The antidote is easy—drink eight to ten glasses of water daily. (A glass or two of juice is fine, but remember that many juices are laden with calories.)

Exercise

Moderate exercise can relieve tension, and tension can add years to your face. A stressed out 20-year-old with 'worry lines' on her forehead can look older than a relaxed and fit 40-year-old.

Maintain Normal Weight

Constant weight loss and gain can rob skin of its flexibility, resulting in sagging skin.

Be Gentle

Don't tug or pull at your face. Cleanse gently with a cotton wool ball or soft facecloth, and pat dry. Loofahs and grainy cleansers are often too rough for many people, and should be used rarely on skin, if at all. People with dry skin should avoid abrasive cleansers altogether.

SUN PROTECTION

As far as your skin is concerned, ultraviolet light is Public Enemy Number One. Although most cases of skin cancer are not serious, some people develop malignant melanoma, which is potentially fatal. And the bad news is that sunscreens and blocks appear not to protect against melanoma. Sun exposure can also accelerate the ageing process—in fact, dermatologists blame as much as 80 per cent of the skin damage associated with ageing on exposure to the sun. Dangerous as the sun may be, I am not

245

suggesting that people spend their days indoors. However, be sure to follow these guidelines:

No Tan is a Good Tan. Until recently, the prevailing philosophy had been that if you generally increased your exposure so that you did not burn, and wore a good sunscreen, it was possible to tan safely. We now know that there is no such thing as a good tan. Tanning is the body's response to injury and should be avoided.

Avoid Peak Exposure. Do as my friend the dermatologist does: during the summer he runs for shelter between the hours of 10 a.m. and 2 p.m. when the sun is at its strongest. Confine your outdoor activities to early morning or late afternoon.

Check Your Medication. Some medication, such as tetracycline or Retin-A, or even some diuretics, can increase sensitivity to the sun. If you are taking any medication, be sure to consult your doctor before spending time out of doors.

Wear Sunscreen. Wear a sunscreen every day with a sun protection factor (SPF) of 15. Sunscreens come as high as SPF 50, but many people may find these stronger screens irritating. The SPF means that you can stay out in the sun that many times longer with the sunscreen on without burning than without it. Even if you use a waterproof sunscreen, always reapply after swimming or sweating, or at least every two hours. Apply your sunscreen at least a half an hour before going out in the sun—it takes time to soak into the skin.

A good sunscreen should protect against both UVA and UVB rays. UVB rays can cause wrinkling and damage to your skin. UVA rays, once believed to be safe, have also been shown to cause significant skin damage. For the best protection, use a broad spectrum sunscreen that can reflect UV rays as well as absorb them. For example, some sunscreens contain titanium dioxide, a chemical that reflects UV light off the skin and is often used in so-called 'chemical free' sunscreens. (In reality, no sunscreen is chemical free; rather, the active ingredient sits on top of the skin and does not get absorbed.)

Many people may be allergic to some of the ingredients used in sunscreens. For example, PABA (para-aminobenzoic acid) a common ingredient, may trigger a rash or irritation in some people. In some cases, reflective sunscreens may be less irritating because they do not interact with the skin. Many brands now claim to be hypoallergenic, which means they are less prone to cause a rash or irritation. Others claim to be noncomedogenic or nonacnegenic, which means that they are less likely to clog pores. No matter what the manufacturer may claim, if you are sensitive to skin products in general, be sure to try out a sunscreen on a small area of skin before using it all over your body. If the area remains irritation-free for 24 hours, the product is probably safe for you. If in doubt, consult your doctor.

If your skin dries out in the sun, be sure to use a sunscreen with a moisturiser. Aloe vera is still my favourite and is included in many sunscreens. It is also good to help heal skin after too much sun exposure.

Of course, it is critical to wear sunscreen in the summer when you are out of doors more, but many dermatologists advise their patients to use sunscreens all year round, at least on their faces— indeed, many brands of make-up now include SPF protection. Using a foundation with a sunscreen is an easy way to make sure that your face is protected daily.

Bronzers. There are several products on the market that can help you tan without ever setting foot in the sun. These contain dehydroxyacetone which I am told is harmless, but I am always reluctant to recommend chemicals, particularly if they have not been in use for that long a time. However, if you want a healthy glow, there is nothing wrong with using one of the new skin bronzers that are being marketed by several cosmetics companies. Although bronzers can make you look as if you have just stepped off the beach, they are a lot kinder to your skin. Some even offer UV protection.

Protective Clothing. A dark T-shirt or trousers will help protect against ultraviolet rays, and special SPF outdoor clothing is also available from some sportswear shops or mail order companies.

Sunglasses. Sunglasses can prevent squinting, which can promote crows' feet and fine lines around the eyes. (They can also protect against cataracts.) Be sure to buy sunglasses that offer UV protection.

DRY SKIN

Dry, itchy skin is a common complaint among older people, especially in the winter. It is caused by a reduction in sebum, an oil that forms a protective coating on the skin, thus sealing in moisture. Although you cannot replace lost moisture (as some advertisements for skin care products would have you believe) you can bolster the body's own protective seal by using products that reduce water loss from the skin's surface. There are numerous creams and potions on the market that can help seal in moisture. I recommend using fragrance-free, allergy-tested products which are relatively inexpensive and work quite well for people with mild cases of dry skin. Plain old petroleum jelly can work wonders on hands and feet, and aloe vera creams and lotions, and jojoba oil (from the jojoba plant) are also excellent for dry skin and quite reasonably priced. In severe cases your doctor may prescribe a more potent moisturiser.

There are several 'new generation' moisturisers on the market which contain various fancy-sounding compounds. Basically, despite the hype, these products are similar to traditional moisturisers in that they seal in moisture, although some may work better than others. There is a wide range of prices among these product lines, and some of the cheaper ones sold by your local chemist may be just as effective as some of the products sold in fancy department stores.

Avoid using harsh soaps—soap free cleansers work well and are far less irritating for most people. Don't bathe or shower in very hot water. An oatmeal bath can offer instant relief for dry skin.

Dry heat in particular may sap needed moisture from your skin. Turn off the heat and wear a jersey, or use a humidifier which could reduce dryness. However, make sure that you are scrupulous about maintaining and cleaning the humidifier because it could be a breeding ground for bacteria and fungi.

For severe dry skin, try taking one linseed oil capsule three times daily. Within a month, you should see softer, more supple skin.

COSMECEUTICALS

'Cosmeceuticals' refers to a new breed of skin products that offer both therapeutic and cosmetic benefits. Unlike traditional make-ups that merely covered up flaws and blemishes, cosmeceuticals contain biologically active ingredients that (according to their manufacturers) actually change the quality of the skin. Even sceptics agree that these new breeds of skin cream do have an effect on the outer layers of skin, at least temporarily. Tretonin (marketed as Retin-A), was the first cosmeceutical. Although originally designed to treat acne, dermatologists noticed that it appeared to erase fine lines, and peeled off the top layer of skin, leaving a pinkish, healthy glow. However, many patients found Retin-A very irritating, and it also caused excessive sun-sensitivity. Nevertheless, Retin-A is now one of the most prescribed medications in the world. There is a host of other cosmeceuticals on the market, notably Vitamin A derivatives, alpha hydroxy acids, salicylic acid and antioxidants.

Retinol, Retinyl Palmitate. These non-prescriptive strength Vitamin A creams are being touted as anti-wrinkle creams without the side effects of Retina-A. Many dermatologists are doubtful whether these creams are strong enough to be effective, but they may work well for some people.

AHAs (which include fruit acid, lactic acid and glycolic acid) are actually exfolients—that is, they peel dead cells off the surface of the skin, making it look smoother and less wrinkled. AHAs also help the skin to maintain moisture. Regular use of AHAs can give the skin a fresh glow and, unlike conventional face creams, they are believed to work below the surface of the skin, dissolving the glue that holds it together. Over-the-counter products contain between two and ten per cent concentrations of AHAs. Dermatologists and plastic surgeons use much stronger concentrations in facial skin peels.

There is a great deal of controversy regarding the effectiveness and safety of these products. Not all dermatologists agree that AHAs are as effective as their manufacturers say they are. Many contend that over-the-counter products are really not strong enough to have any effect, and some dermatologists worry that

249

the skin will eventually adjust to the AHA, and that higher and higher concentrations may be required for any noticeable change. As things are now, many people find that even low levels can be irritating. Some doctors also express concern about potential hazards resulting from the long-term use of these new products. They point out that no one knows what if any ill effects could arise from several decades of use. What is even more alarming is that some beauty salons offer AHA treatments using concentrations of up to 70 per cent, which could well cause damage. My advice is, proceed with caution. I don't believe that using the lower concentrations of AHAs (under ten per cent) will be harmful so long as you can tolerate them. If you develop any irritation, discontinue the product. Unless the label says otherwise, do not apply an AHA product near the eyes.

Salicylic Acid. Similar to AHAs, salicylic acid also sloughs away dead cells and promotes cell turnover (the production of new cells). Salicylic acid may be less irritating for some people, and some dermatologists believe that it is somewhat more effective. At least one study suggested that it promoted faster cell regeneration than AHAs.

Antioxidants. Antioxidants are substances that can prevent damage caused by free radicals, unstable oxygen molecules which can destroy healthy cells. Ultraviolet light in particular can wreak havoc on the skin by creating more of these troublesome free radicals. Antioxidant vitamins such as beta-carotene, E and C, and superoxide dismutase (SOD), an antioxidant enzyme which is produced by the body, are included in many skin care products. Although not everyone is convinced of the effectiveness of the external use of antioxidants, it seems possible that they may help to prevent UV damage. Some researchers also believe that antioxidant creams may help to prevent skin cancer.

Resources

The following organisations can provide information, help and advice. Many offer support services by means of self-help groups and have a network of local groups. Ask them if there is one in your area. Leaflets and books are available in many cases, and some organisations publish a regular magazine for members.

GENERAL

Age Concern (England), Astral House, 1268 London Road, Norbury, London SW16 4ER. (Tel: 0181 679 8000)

Age Concern (Scotland), 54a Fountainbridge, Edinburgh EH3 9PT. (Tel: 0131 228 5656)

Age Concern (Wales), 1 Cathedral Road, Transport House, 4th Floor, Cardiff, South Glamorgan CF1 9SD. (Tel: 01222 371821/371566)

Age Concern (Northern Ireland), 3 Lower Crescent, Belfast BT7 1NR. (Tel: 01232 245729)

British Association for Service to the Elderly (BASE), 119 Hassell Street, Newcastle-under-Lyme, Staffordshire ST5 1AX. (Tel: 01782 661033)

Centre for Policy on Ageing, 25–31 Ironmonger Row, London EC1V 3QP. (Tel: 0171 253 1787)

Counsel and Care for the Elderly, Twyman House, 16 Bonny Street, London NW1 9LR. (Tel: 0171 485 1550)

Help the Aged, St James's Walk, London EC1R OBE. (Tel: 0171 253 0253. SeniorLine: 0800 289404)

ALTERNATIVE THERAPIES

The Bach Flower Remedies, The Bach Centre, Mount Vernon, Sotwell, Wallingford, Oxon. OX10 OPZ. (Tel: 01491 34678). For advice and information.

The Bach Flower Remedies, Unit 6, Suffolk Way, Abingdon, Oxon. OX14 5JX. (Tel: 01235 550086). For orders for remedies and books.

British Homoeopathic Association, 27a Devonshire Street, London W1N 1RJ. (Tel: 0171 935 2163)

International Federation of Aromatherapists, Royal Masonic Hospital, Ravenscourt Park, London W6 OTN. (Tel: 0181 846 8066)

National Institute of Medical Herbalists, 9 Palace Gate, Exeter, Devon EX1 1JA. (Tel: 01392 426022)

Institute of Chinese Medicine, 44 Chandos Place, London WC2N 4HS. (Tel: 0171 836 5220)

The UK T'ai Chi Association, PO Box 159, Bromley, Kent BR1 3XX.

ARTHRITIS

Arthritis Care, 18 Stephenson Way, London NW1 2HD. (Tel: 0171 916 1500. Helpline: 0800 289170)

Arthritis and Rheumatism Research Council, PO Box 177, Chesterfield S41 7TQ. (Tel: 01246 558033)

BRAIN FUNCTION

Action for Dysphasic Adults (ADA), 1 Royal Street, London SE1 7LL. (Tel: 0171 261 9572)

Alzheimer's Disease Society, Gordon House, 10 Greencoat Place, London SW1P 1PH. (Tel: 0171 306 0606. Information and advice: 0171 306 0833)

British Epilepsy Association, Anstey House, 40 Hanover Square, Leeds LS3 1BE. (Tel: 0113 2439393. Advice: 0113 2089599)

College of Speech and Language Therapists, 7 Bath Place, Rivington Street, London EC2A 3DR. (Tel: 0171 613 3855)

MIND, 20–22 Harley Street, London W1N 2ED. (Tel: 0171 637 0741).

Parkinson's Disease Society, 12 Upper Woburn Place, London WC1H OEP. (Tel: 0171 383 3513)

The Stroke Association, CHSA House, Whitecross Street, London EC1Y 8JJ. (Tel: 0171 490 7999)

CANCER

British Association of Cancer United Patients (BACUP), Cancer Information Service, 3 Bath Place, London EC2A 3JR. (Tel: 0171 613 2121)

CancerLink Ltd, 17 Britannia Street, London WC1X 9JN. (Tel: 0171 833 2451)

Cancer Prevention Research Trust, 36 Roehampton Vale, London SW15 3SF. (Tel: 0181 789 1262)

Cancer Relief Macmillan Fund, 15 Britten Street, London SW3 3TZ. (Tel: 0171 353 7811)

Cancer Research Campaign, 6–10 Cambridge Terrace, London NW1 4JL (Tel: 0171 2244 1333)

Cancer You Are Not Alone (CYANA), 31 Church Road, London E12 6AD. (Tel: 0181 553 0333)

Imperial Cancer Research Fund, 44 Lincolns Inn Fields, London WC2A 3PX. (Tel: 0171 242 0200)

DIABETES

British Diabetic Association, 10 Queen Anne Street, London W1M OBD. (Tel: 0171 323 1531)

HEARING

British Deaf Association, 38 Victoria Place, Carlisle, Cumbria CA1 1HU. (Tel: 01228 48844)

British Society of Hearing Therapists, The Leicester Royal

Infirmary, Leicester LE1 5WW. (Tel: 0116 2541414 ext. 55778)

British Tinnitus Association, 14–18 West Bar Green, Sheffield SA1 2DA. (Tel: 0114 2796600)

Hearing Concern: The British Association of the Hard of Hearing, 7–11 Armstrong Road, London W3 7JL. (Tel: 0181 743 1110)

National Association of Deafened People, Longacre, Horsleys Green, High Wycombe, Buckinghamshire HP14 3UX.

The Royal National Institute for Deaf People (RNID), 105 Gower Street, London WC1E 6AH. (0171 387 8033. Information: 0800 413 114)

HEART

The British Heart Foundation, 14 Fitzhardinge Street, London W1H 4DH. (Tel: 0171 935 0185)

Coronary Artery Disease Association, Tavistock House North, Tavistock Square, London WC1H 9HP. (Tel: 0171 387 9779)

The Coronary Prevention Group, Plantation House, Fenchurch Street, London EC3M 3DX. (Tel: 0171 626 4844)

NUTRITION AND HEALTH

British Association for Nutritional Therapy, PO Box 3AP, London W1A 3AP. (Tel: 0171 436 8532)

British Society for Nutritional Medicine, 72 Main Street, Osgathorpe, Leics. LE12 9TA.

Institute for Optimum Nutrition, 5 Jerdan Place, London SW6 1BE. (Tel: 0171 385 7984)

The Nutrition Society, 10 Cambridge Court, Shepherds Bush Road, London W12 7NG. (Tel: 0171 602 0228)

OSTEOPOROSIS

Osteoporosis Society, PO Box 10, Radstock, Bath, Avon BA3 3YB. (Tel: 01761 432472)

SIGHT

National Deaf-Blind League, 18 Rainbow Court, Paston Ridings, Peterborough PE4 6UP. (Tel: 01733 73511)

Partially Sighted Society, 62 Salusbury Road, London NW6 6NP. (Tel: 0171 372 1551)

The Royal National Institute for the Blind (RNIB), 224 Great Portland Street, London W1N 6AA. (Tel: 0171 388 1266)

HERBALISTS AND HEALTH SUPPLEMENTS

Baldwin & Co., 173 Walworth Road, London SE17 1RN. (Tel: 0171 703 5550)

Chinese Herbal Health Consultants, 44–46 Buckingham Palace Road, London SW1. (Tel: 0171 828 9836)

Culpepper Ltd., 21 Bruton Street, London W1X 7DA. (Tel: 0171 629 4559)

Health Perception Ltd., Winkfield Row, Berkshire RG12 8NY. (Tel: 01344 890115)

The Herb Society, 134 Buckingham Palace Road, London SW1W 9SA. (Tel: 0171 823 5583)

Larkhall Green Farm, 225 Putney Bridge Road, London SW15 2PY. (Tel: 0181 874 1130)

Selected Bibliography

Acoustic Neuroma Association Notes, No. 36, December 1990.

Aldercreutz, Herman. 'Plasma Concentrations of Phyto-Oestrogens in Japanese Men.' *The Lancet*, 342:1209–1210, November 13, 1993.

—— 'Lignans and Phytoestrogens: Possible Protective Role in Cancer.' *Frontiers of Gastrointestinal Research*, 14:165–176, 1988.

Aldercreutz, H., Hamalainen, E., Gorbach, S., and Goldin, B. 'Dietary Phyto-oestrogens and the Manopause in Japan.' *The Lancet*, 339:1233, May 16, 1992.

Anderson, James W. 'Dietary Fiber and Diabetes.' *Journal of the American Dietetic Association*. 87(9): September 1987.

'A Test to Take (and not to take) for colon cancer.' University of California at Berkeley Wellness Letter, 9(12): September 1993.

al-Hindawa MK; al-Khafaji, S.H.; Abdul-Nabi, M.H. *Journal of Ethnopharmacology*. 37(2):113–116, September 1992.

'Aloe Update.' *The Lawrence Review of Natural Products*. 3(21): November 15, 1982.

Anderson, James W. *The HCF Guide Book*. HCF Diabetes Foundation, Lexington, Kentucky, 1987.

Armstrong, S.M. and Redman, J.R. 'Melatonin: A Chronobiotic with Anti-Aging Properties.' *Medical Hypotheses*, 43:300–309, 1991.

'Aspirin as a Therapeutic Agent in Cardiovascular Disease.' American Heart Association. Dallas, Tx., 1993.

Balch, James F. and Baclh, Phyllis, A. *Prescription for Nutritional Healing*. Garden City, New York, Avery Publishing Group, 1990.

Barbul, Adrian, M.D.; Sisto, Donato, A.; Wasserkrug, Hannah

L., *et al.* 'Arginine Stimulates Lymphocyte Immune Response in Healthy Human Beings.' *Surgery*, 90(1):244–251, 1981.

'Be Your Best: Nutrition After Fifty.' American Institute for Cancer Research, Washington, D.C., 1988.

'Beyond Deficiency: New Views on the Function and Health Effects of Vitamins.' The New York Academy of Sciences, February 9–12, 1992. Abstracts.

Bitterman, Wilhelm, A., Farhadian, Haim., *et al.* 'Environmental and Nutritional Factors Significantly Associated with Cancer of the Urinary Tract Among Different Ethnic Groups.' *Urologic Clinics of North America*, 18(3): August 1991.

Bland, Jeffrey. *Bioflavonoids: The Friends and Helpers of Vitamin C in Many Hard-to-Treat Ailments*. New Canaan, Conn.: Keats Publishing Inc., 1984.

Block, Gladys; Henson, Donald E.; Levine, Mark. eds. 'Ascorbic Acid: Biologic Functions and Relation to Cancer.' Proceedings of the National Institutes of Health, Bethesda, Md. September 10–12, 1990. *The American Journal of Clinical Nutrition*, Supplement to 54(6): December 1991.

'Blocking Skin Cancer Through Diet?' *Tufts University Diet and Nutrition Letter*, 12(5): July 1994.

Blumenthal, Mark. 'Echinacea Highlighted as Cold and Flu Remedy.' *Herbalgram*, No. 29, 8–9, 1993.

'Borage Seed Oil and Evening Primrose Oil May Relieve Arthritis Pain and Swelling.' *Environmental Nutrition*, March 1994.

Borum, Peggy, R. 'Carnitine.' *Annual Review in Nutrition*, 3:233–259, 1983.

Bowman, Barbara. 'Acetyl-Carnitine and Alzheimer's Disease.' *Nutrition Reviews*, 50(5).

Bradlow, H. Leon and Michnovicz, Jon. 'A New Approach to the prevention of Breast Cancer.' *Proceedings of the Royal Society of Edinburgh*, 95B:77–86, 1989.

Brody, Jane. 'Folic Acid Emerges as a Nutritional Star.' *The New York Times*, March 1, 1994.

Bunce, George Edwin. 'Nutritional Factors in Cataract.' *Annual Review of Nutrition*, 10:233–254, 1990.

'. . . But Study of Women Finds Iron May Contribute to Higher

Coronary Disease Risk.' News from the American Heart Association, Dallas, Texas, June 13, 1994.

Butterworth, C.E., Hatch, Kenneth D., Macaluso, Maurizio, *et al.* 'Folate Deficiency and Cervical Dysplasia.' *JAMA*, 267(4): January 22–29, 1992.

Butrin, Ritva B., Clifford, Carolyn, Lanza, Elaine. 'NCI Dietary Guidelines: rationale.' *American Journal of Clinical Nutrition*, 48:888–895, 1988.

Cancer Facts and Figures – 1993. American Cancer Society. Atlanta, Ga, 1993.

Caragay, Alegria B. 'Cancer-Preventive Foods and Ingredients.' *Food Technology*, 46(4):65–68, April 1992.

Castleman, Michael. 'Red Pepper is Hot!' *Medical Selfcare*, 68–69, September/October 1989.

Cerda, J.J., Robbins, F.L., Burgin, C.W. *et al.* 'The Effects of Grapefruit Pectin on Patients at Risk for Coronary Heart Disease Without Altering Diet or Lifestyle.' *Clinical Cardiology*, 11(9):589–594, September 1988.

Chen, K.J. and Chen, K. 'Ischaemic Stroke Treated with Ligusticum Chuanxiong.' *Chinese Medical Journal*, 105(10):870–873, October 1992.

Chinthalapally, Rao V., Desai, Dhimant, Simi, Barbara, *et al.* 'Inhibitory Effect of Caffeic Acid Esters on Azoxymethane-induced Biochemical Changes and Aberrant Crypt Foci Formation in Rat Colon.' *Cancer Research*, 53:4182–4188, September 15, 1993.

'Chronic Stress is Directly Linked to Premature Aging of the Brain.' *Research Bulletin*, National Institute on Aging, Bethesda, Md. October 1991.

Cutler, Richard G. 'Antioxidants and Aging.' *American Journal of Clinical Nutrition*, 53:373S–379S, 1991.

Darlington, L. Gail. 'Dietary Therapy for Arthritis.' *Rheumatic Disease Clinics of North America*, 17(2):273–285, May 1991.

Darlington, L.G., Ramsey, S.W. 'Clinical Review: Review of Dietary Therapy for Rheumatoid Arthritis.' *British Journal of Rheumatology*, 32:507–514, 1993.

Devi, P.U., Sharada, A.C., Solomon, F.E., Kamath, M.S. 'In vivo inhibitory effect of *Withania somnifera* (Ashwagandha) on a transplantable mouse tumour, Sarcoma 180.' *Indian Journal Experimental Biology*, 30(3):169–172, March 1992.

Diet and Cancer. American Institute for Cancer Research, Information Series. Washington, D.C., 1992.

Diet, Nutrition, and Prostate Cancer. American Institute for Cancer Research, Information Series. Washington, D.C., 1991.

'Dizziness, Hope Through Research.' U.S. Department of Health and Human Services, National Institutes of Health, Bethesda, Md., September 1986.

'Do Monounsaturated Fats and Vitamin E Provide Double-Barrelled Protection Against Coronary Ills?' News from the American Heart Association, Dallas, Texas, April 11, 1994.

Dorgan, Joanne F., Schatzkin, Arthur. 'Antioxidant Micronutrients in Cancer Prevention.' *Nutrition and Cancer*, 5(1):43–61.

Duke, James A. 'An Herb a Day: Clubmoss, alias Lycopodium alias Huperzia.' *Business of Herbs*, January/February 1989.

Elegbede, J.A., Elson, C.E., Tanner, M.A. *et al.* 'Regression of Rat Primary Mammary Tumors Following Dietary d-Limonene.' *Journal of the National Cancer Institute*, 76(2):323–325, February 1986.

'Estrogen and Alzheimer's.' *Harvard Women's Health Watch*, 1(11): July 1994.

Evans, Williams J. 'Exercise, Nutrition and Aging.' Symposium: Nutrition and Exercise, American Institute of Nutrition, 1992.

'Exercise and Arthritis: The Importance of a Regular Program.' *UC Berkeley Wellness Letter*, April 1994.

'Exercise in 90-Year-Olds Increases Muscle Strength and Mobility.' National Institute on Aging Research Bulletin, Bethesda, Md., September 3, 1990.

Fackelmann, K.A. 'Chicken Cartilage Soothes Aching Joints.' *Science News*, 144:198, September 25, 1993.

—— 'Nutrients May Prevent Blinding Disease.' *Science News*, 145: September 12, 1994.

—— 'Do EMFs Pose Breast Cancer Risk?' *Science News*, 145: June 18, 1994.

'Facts and Fiction About Memory Aging: A Quantitative

Integration of Research Findings.' *Journal of Gerontology*, 48(4):157–171, 1993.

'Facts on Prostate Cancer.' American Cancer Society, 1988.

Feldman, Henry A., Goldstein, Irwin, Hatzichristou, Dimitrios *et al.* 'Impotence and its Medical and Psychosocial Correlates: Results of the Massachusetts Male Aging Study.' *Journal of Urology*, 151:54–61, January 1994.

Fiatarone, Maria, O'Neill, Evelyn, F., Ryan, Nancy Doyle. 'Exercise Training and Nutritional Supplementation for Physical Frailty in Very Elderly People.' *New England Journal of Medicine*, 330(25):June 23, 1994.

'Flax Facts.' *Journal of the National Cancer Institute*, 83(15):1050–1052, September 7, 1991.

Food and Nutrition, Research Briefs. United States Department of Agriculture, January–March 1993.

Food and Nutrition, Research Briefs. United States Department of Agriculture, July–September 1993.

Garland, Cedric F., Garland, Frank, C. and Gorham, Edward D. 'Can Colon Cancer Incidence and Death Rates be Reduced with Calcium and Vitamin D?' *American Journal of Clinical Nutrition*, 54:193S–201S, 1991.

'Garlic Fights Nitrosamine Formation . . . as do Tomatoes, and other Produce.' *Science News*, 145:190, 1994.

'Ginger and Atractylodes as an Anti-inflammatory.' *Herbalgram*, No. 29, 19, 1993.

Giovannucci, Edward, Rimm, Eric B., Colditz, G. 'A Prospective Study of Dietary Fat and Risk of Prostate Cancer.' *Journal of the National Cancer Institute*, 85(19): October 16, 1993.

Graf, Ernst and Eaton, John W. 'Antioxidant Functions of Phytic Acid.' *Free Radical Biology and Medicine*, 8:61–69, 1990.

Hackman, Robert M. 'Palm Oil Carotene: An Exciting New Innovation in Nutrition Supplementation.' *Whole Foods*, December 1993.

Heart and Stroke Facts. The American Heart Association, Dallas, Tx. 1994.

Heimburger, D.C., Alexander, C.B., Birch, R. *et al.* 'Improvement in Bronchial Squamous Metaplasia in Smokers Treated with Folate and Vitamin B12. Report of a Preliminary

Randomized, Double-Blind Intervention Trial.' *JAMA*, 259(10):1525–1530, March 11, 1988.

'Herbs and Spices May be Barrier Against Cancer, Heart Disease.' *Environmental Nutrition*, 16(6):June 1993.

Hobbs, Christopher and Foster, Steven. 'Hawthorne: A Literature Review.' *Herbalgram*. No. 22, 19–33, Spring 1990.

Hocman, Gabriel. 'Prevention of Cancer: Vegetables and Plants.' *Comp. Biochem. Physiol.*, 93B(2):201–212, 1989.

Hodge, Marie. 'Immunity "Breakthrough": The 6000-Year-Old Rx.' *Longevity*, January 1993.

Horwitt, Max K. 'Therapeutic Uses of Vitamin E.' *Resident and Staff Physician*, 38–46, December 1982.

—— 'How Men Stay Young.' Emmaus, Pa.: Rodale Press, 1991.

Horwitz, Crystal, and Walker, Alexander R.P. 'Lignans—Additional Benefits From Fibre?' *Nutrition and Cancer*, 6(2):1984.

'Improved Physician/Patient Communication Can Minimise Some Drug Side Effects.' *Research Bulletin*, National Institute on Aging, Bethesda: January 30, 1989.

'In vino veritas—and something for your heat.' *Heartstyle*, 4(3):Summer 1994.

Jaakkolla, K., Lahteenmaki, J. *et al.* 'Treatment with Antioxidant and Other Nutrients in Combination with Chemotherapy and Irradiation in Patients with Small-Cell Lung Cancer.' *Anticancer Research*, 12:599–606, 1992.

Jain, Adesh K., Vargas, Ramon, Gotzkowsky, Sandra *et al.* 'Can Garlic Reduce Levels of Serum Lipids? A Controlled Clinical Study.' *American Journal of Medicine*, 94:632–635, June 1993.

Johnson, Kathleen, and Kligman, Evan W. 'Preventive Nutrition: An "Optimal" Diet for Older Adults.' *Geriatrics*, 47(10):56–60.

Johnston, Carol S., Meyer, Claudia, and Srilakshmi, J.C. 'Vitamin C Elevates Red Blood Cell Gluathione in Healthy Adults.' *American Journal of Clinical Nutrition*, 58:103–105, 1993.

Joosten, Etienne, van der Ber, Annelise, Riezler, Reiner *et al.*

'Metabolic Evidence that Deficiencies of Vitamin B-12 (cobalamin), Folate, and Vitamin B-6 Occur Commonly in Elderly People.' *American Journal of Clinical Nutrition,* 58:468–476, 1993.

Kamikawa, Todashi, Kobayashi, Akira, Yamashita, Tetsuo *et al.,* 'Effects of Coenzyme Q10 on Exercise Tolerance in Chronic Stable Angina Pectoris.' *American Journal of Cardiology,* 56:247–251, 1985.

Khachaturian, Zaven S. 'Calcium and the Aging Brain: Upsetting a Delicate Balance?' *Geriatrics,* 46(6):1991.

Khan, A., Bryden, N.A., Polansky, M.M., Anderson R.A. 'Insulin Potentiating Factor and Chromium Content of Selected Foods and Spices.' *Biologic Trace Element Research,* 24(3):183–188, March 1990.

Kravitz, Howard, M., Sabelli, Hector C., Fawcett, Jan. 'Dietary Supplements of Phenylalanine and Other Amino Acid Precursors of Brain Neuroamines in the Treatment of Depressive Disorders.' *Journal of the AOA,* 84(1): Supplement, September 1984.

Kune, Gabriel, Bannerman, Susan, Field, Barry. 'Diet, Alcohol, Smoking, Serum B-Carotene, and Vitamin A in Male Non-melanocytic Skin Cancer Patients and Controls.' *Nutrition and Cancer,* 18(3):237–244, 1992.

Lee, H.P., Gourley, L., Duffy, S.W. *et al.* 'Dietary Effects on Breast-Cancer Risk in Singapore.' *The Lancet,* 337, 1197–1200, May 18, 1991.

Leighton, Terrance, Ginther, Charles, Fluss, Larry. 'The Distribution of Quercetin and Quercetin Glycosides in Vegetable Components of the Human Diet.' Paper delivered at the Royal Society of Chemistry Conference, September 1992.

Lipkin, Richard. 'Wine's Chemical Secrets.' *Science News,* 144:264–265, October 23, 1993.

'Long-Distance Runners Double "Dilating" Capacity of Their Coronary Arteries, Researchers Find.' News from the American Heart Association, Dallas, Texas, April 12, 1993.

'Magnesium Lowers Blood Pressure in Some Diabetic Hypertensive.' News from the American Heart Association, Dallas, Texas, September 13, 1990.

'Major Study Reports "Huge" Variance in Heart Rates Among

Nations.' News from the American Heart Association, Dallas, Texas, July 11, 1994.

McCaleb, Rob. 'Astragalus.' Herb Research Foundation, July 30, 1990.

—— 'Bilberry: Microcirculation Enhancer.' Herb Research Foundation, April 29, 1992.

McKeown-Eyssen, Gail E., and Bright-See, Elizabeth. 'Dietary Factors in Colon Cancer: International Relationships.' *Nutrition and Cancer*, 6(3):1984.

McMurdo, Marion E.T., Rennie, Lucy. 'A Controlled Trial of Exercise by Residents of Old People's Homes.' *Age and Ageing*, 22:11–15, 1993.

Meydani, M., Evans, W.J., Handelman, G. *et al.* 'Protective Effect of Vitamin E on Exercise-Induced Oxidative Damage in Young and Older Adults.' *American Journal of Physiology*, 264 (Regulatory Integrative Comp. Physiol. 33):R 992–998, 1993.

Michnovicz, Jon J. and Bradlow, H. Leon. 'Induction of Estradiol Metabolism by Dietary Indole 3-carbinol in Humans.' *Journal of the National Cancer Institute*, 82(11):June 6, 1990.

'Mining for Toxic Minerals Hidden in Our Diets.' *Environmental Nutrition*, 15(3): March 1992.

'Mining for Minerals—Zinc is Worth Its Weight in Gold.' *Environmental Nutrition*, 17(9): September 1994.

Moriguchi, Satori, Mukai, Kiyosha, Hiroaka, Isao *et al.* 'Functional Changes in Human Lymphocytes and Monocytes After In Vitro Incubation with Arginine.' *Nutrition Research*, 7:719–728, 1987.

Nelson, Miriam, E., Fisher, Elizabeth, C., Dilmanian, Avraham, F. 'A 1-year Walking Program and Increased Dietary Calcium in Postmenopausal Women: Effects on Bone.' *American Journal of Clinical Nutrition*, 53:1304–1311, 1991.

Newsome, D.A., Swartz, M., Leone, N.C. *et al.* 'Oral Zinc in Macular Degeneration.' *Archives of Ophthalmology*, 106(2):192–198, February 1988.

'NIH Consensus Development Conference: The Treatment of Sleep Disorders in Older People.' *National Institute on Aging Research Bulletin*, September 3, 1990.

Negri, Eva, Vecchia, Carlo La, Francheschi, Silvia. 'Vegetable and Fruit Consumption and Cancer Risk.' *International Journal of Cancer*, 48:350–354, 1994.

'Niacin: Double-Edged Sword for Lowering Cholesterol.' *Tufts University Diet and Nutrition Letter*, 12(6): August 1994.

Nielson, Forrest H. 'Ultratrace Minerals: Mythical Elixirs or Nutrients of Concern?' *Biologic Association of Medicine of Puerto Rico*, 83:131–133, 1981.

—— 'Studies on the Relationship Between Boron and Magnesium which Possibly Affects the Formation and Maintenance of Bones.' *Magnesium Trace Elements*, 9:61–19, 1990.

Nixon, Daniel W., Winick, Myron, Maher, Michelle. 'Metabolic Efficiency, Energy Intake, and Cancer.' *Cancer Prevention*, 1(3):1991.

'No Need for Kidney Stone Sufferers to Curb Calcium.' *Environmental Nutrition*, September, 1993.

'Noise and Hearing Loss, Consensus Statement.' *NIH Consensus Development Conference*, 8(1): January 22–24, 1990.

Odens, Max. 'Prolongation of the Life Span in Rats.' *Journal of the American Geriatrics Society*, 21(10):450–451, 1973.

'On the Link Between Diet and Gout.' *Tufts University Diet and Nutrition Letter*, 10(9): November 1, 1992.

Packer, Lester. 'Protective Role of Vitamin E in Biologic Systems.' *American Journal of Clinical Nutrition*, 53:1050S–1055S, 1991.

Panush, Richard S. 'Does Food Cause or Cure Arthritis?' *Rheumatic Disease Clinics of North America*, 17(2):259–271, May 1991.

Penn, N.D., Purkins, L., Kelleher, J. *et al.* 'The Effect of Dietary Supplementation with Vitamins A, C, and E on Cell-mediated Immune Function in Elderly Long-stay Patients: A Randomised Controlled Trial.' *Age and Ageing*, 20:169–174, 1991.

Parchellet, J.P., Gali, H.U., Perchellet, E.M. *et al.* 'Antitumor-Promoting Activities of Tannic Acid, Ellagic Acid, and Several Gallic Acid Derivatives in Mouse Skin.' *Basic Life Sciences*, 59:783–801, 1992.

Peto, R., Doll, R., Buckley, J.D. *et al.* 'Can Dietary Beta-Carotene Materially Reduce Human Cancer Rates?' *Nature*, 290:201–207, March 1981.

Press, Raymond I., Geller, Jack, Evans, Gary. 'The Effect of Chromium Picolinate on Serum Cholesterol and Apolipoprotein Fractions in Human Subjects.' *The Western Journal of Medicine*, 152(1):41–45, January 1990.

'Preventing Wintertime Bone Loss: Effect of Vitamin D Supplementation in Healthy Postmenopausal Women.' *Nutrition Reviews*, 50(2):52–54.

'Preventive Nutrition: Disease-Specific Dietary Interventions for Older Adults.' *Geriatrics*, 47(11):39–49, November 1992.

'Prostate Cancer and Red Meat.' *UC Berkeley Wellness Letter*, February 1994.

Pryor, William A. 'Can Vitamin E Protect Humans Against the Pathological Effects of Ozone in Smog?' *American Journal of Clinical Nutrition*, 53:702–722, 1991.

'Pumping Immunity.' *Nutrition Action Healthletter*, April 1993.

Raloff, Janet. 'Hearty Vitamins: Sparing Arteries With Megadose Supplements.' *Science News*, 142:78, 1991.

Reiger, Martin M. 'Oxidative reactions in and on skin: mechanism and prevention.' Allured Publishing Corporation, December 1993.

Research Briefs, U.S. Department of Agriculture, Greenbelt, Md., April–June 1993.

Research Bulletin, National Institute on Aging, Bethesda, Md., February 20, 1990.

—— April 1991.

—— July 1991.

—— October 1991.

—— August 1992.

—— November 1992.

'Reviving Your Taste Buds When Taste and Smell Wane.' *Environmental Nutrition*, February 1993.

Risch, Harvey A., Meera Jain, N. Won Choi *et al.* 'Dietary Factors and the Incidence of Cancer of the Stomach.' *American Journal of Epidemiology*, 122(6):1985.

Robertson, James McD., Donner, Allan P., Trevithick, John R. 'A Possible Role for Vitamins C and E in Cataract Prevention.' *American Journal of Clinical Nutrition*, 53:346S–351S, 1991.

Roe, Daphne, A. 'Overview of Effects of Aging on Nutrition.'

Clinics in Geriatric Medicine, 6(2):319–334, May 1990.

Roebothan, Barbara Vera, Chandra, Ranja Kumar. 'Relationship between Nutritional Status and Immune Function of Elderly People.' *Age and Ageing*, 23:49–53, 1994.

Rose, David P. 'Diet, Hormones and Cancer.' *Annual Review of Public Health*, 14:1–17, 1993.

—— 'Dietary Fiber, Phytoestrogens, and Breast Cancer.' *Nutrition*, 8(1):47–51, January/February 1992.

Rosenberg, Irwin H. and Miller, Joshua W. 'Nutritional Factors in Physical and Cognitive Function of Elderly People.' *American Journal of Clinical Nutrition*, 55:1237S–1243S, 1992.

Rusting, Ricki L. 'Why Do We Age?' *Scientific American*, 131–141, December, 1992.

Sandyk, Reuven. 'Possible Role of Pineal Melatonin in the Mechanisms of Aging.' *International Journal of Neuroscience*, 52:85–92, 1990.

Schardt, David. 'Alzheimer's in the Family.' *Nutrition Action Healthletter*, June 1994.

Schlant, Robert C. 'Alcohol and the Cardiovascular System.' *Journal of the American Medical Association*, 264(3):377–381.

Schmidt, Karlheinz. 'Antioxidant vitamins and B-carotene: effects on immunocompetance.' *American Journal of Clinical Nutrition*, 53:383S–385S, 1991.

Selkoe, Dennis J. 'Aging Brain, Aging Mind. Structural and Chemical Changes.' *Scientific American*, 267(3):September 1992.

'Seedy Remedy for Rheumatoid Arthritis?' *Science News*, 144:302, November 6, 1993.

Shephard, Roy J. 'Exercise and Aging: Extending Independence in Older Adults.' *Geriatrics*, 48(5): May 1993.

Sharma, Om P., Adlercreutz, Herman, Strandberg, John D. *et al.* 'Soy of Dietary Source Plays a Preventive Role Against the Pathogenesis of Prostatitis.' *Journal Steroid Biochemical Molecular Biology*, 43(65):557–564, 1992.

Siani, Alfonso, Strazzullo, Pasquale, Giacco, Angela, *et al.* 'Increasing the Dietary Potassium Intake Reduces the Need for Antihypertensive Medication.' *Annals of Internal Medicine*, 115:753–759, 1991.

Simopoulos, Artermis, P. 'Omega-3 Fatty Acids in Health and Disease and in Growth and Development.' *American Journal of Clinical Nutrition*, 54:438–463, 1991.

Smigel, Kara. 'Vitamin E Moves on Stage in Cancer Prevention Studies.' *Journal of the National Cancer Institute*, 84(13): July 1, 1992.

Snyder, Jessica. 'Solving the Alzheimer's Jigsaw.' *Longevity*, January 1992.

Soni, K.B., Rajan, A., Kuttan, R. 'Reversal of Aflatoxin Induced Liver Damage by Turmeric and Curcumin.' *Cancer Letter*, 66(2):115–121, September 30, 1992.

'Staying Physically Active May Help to Stave Off Blood Vessel Ills, Two New Studies Suggest.' News from the American Heart Association, 33rd Annual Conference on Cardiovascular Disease Epidemiology and Prevention, *Abstracts* 17, 18.

Stern, Yaakov, Gurland, Barry *et al.* 'Influence of Education and Occupation on the Incidence of Alzheimer's Disease. *Journal of the American Medical Association*, 271(13): April 6, 1994.

Tanaka, T., Kojima, T., Kawamori, T. *et al.* 'Inhibition of 4-nitroquinoline-1-oxide-induced rat tongue carcinogenesis by the naturally occurring plant phenolics caffeic, ellagic, chlorogenic and ferrulic acids.' *Carcinogenesis*, 14(7):1321–1325, July 1993.

Teas, Jane. 'The Consumption of Seaweed as a Protective Factor in the Etiology of Breast Cancer.' *Medical Hypotheses*, 7:601–613, 1981.

Teel, R.W. and Castonguay, A. 'Antimutagenic effects of polyphenolic compounds.' *Cancer Letter*, 66(2):107–113, September 30, 1992.

'The Food Guide Pyramid.' Human Nutrition Service, USDA, *Home and Garden Bulletin* No. 252, August, 1992.

Thun, Michael J., Calle, Eugenia E., Namboordiri, Mohan, M. *et al.* 'Risk Factors for Fatal Colon Cancer in a Large Prospective Study.' *Journal of the National Cancer Institute*, 84(19): October 7, 1992.

'Triglycerides finally unmasked as "bad actor" in coronary artery disease drama, researchers say.' News from the American Heart Association, Dallas, Texas, July 1994.

Troll, Walter, Kennedy, Ann R. (eds). 'Workshop Report from

the Division of Cancer Etiology, National Cancer Institute, National Institutes of Health. Protease Inhibitors as Cancer Chemopreventive Agents.' *Cancer Research*, 49:499–502, January 15, 1989.

Tucker, Don M., Penland, James G., Sandstead, Harold *et al.* 'Nutrition Status and Brain Function in Aging.' *American Journal of Clinical Nutrition*, 52:93–102, 1990.

'23-Year Study of Middle-Aged Men in Hawaii Confirms: Physical Activity Will Lower Risk of Heart Disease.' News from the American Heart Association, Dallas, Texas, June 13, 1994.

United States Department of Agriculture, Human Nutrition Research Center on Aging at Tufts University, Research Program Description.

Varma, Shambhu, D. 'Scientific Basis for Medical Therapy of Cataracts by Antioxidants.' *American Journal of Clinical Nutrition*, 53:335–345S, 1991.

'Vitamin B6 and Immune Function in the Elderly and HIV-seropositive Subjects.' *Nutrition Reviews*, 50(5):145–147, May 1992.

'Vitamin E May Guard Against Artery Blockage by LDL.' *Heartstyle*, Fall 1993.

'Vitamin E Supplementation Enhances Immune Response in the Elderly.' *Nutrition Reviews*, 50(3):85–87, March 1992.

Walsh, Nicolas E., Ramamurthy, Somayaji, Schoenfield, Lawrence, Hoffman, Joan. 'Analgesic Effectiveness of D-Phenylalanine in Chronic Pain Patients.' *Archives of Physical Medicine Rehabilitation*, 67:436–439, July 1986.

Wei-Hua, Lu, Shou, Jiang, Tang, Xi-Can. 'Improving Effect of Huperzine A on Discrimination Performance in Aged Rats and Adult Rats with Experimental Cognitive Impairment.' *Acta Pharmacologica Sinica*, 1:11–15, January 1988.

Wuethrich, B. 'Higher Risk of Alzheimer's Linked to Gene.' *Science News*, 144: August 14, 1993.

You, W.C., Blot, W.J., Chang, Y.S. *et al.* 'Allium Vegetables and the Reduced Risk of Stomach Cancer.' *Journal of the National Cancer Institute*, 81(2):162–164, 1989.

Znaiden, Alex. 'The Science Behind Successful New Skin Care Products.' *Avanstar Communications*, January 1994.

Ziegler, Regina G. 'Vegetables, Fruits and Carotenoids and the

Risk of Cancer.' *American Journal of Clinical Nutrition*, 53:251S–259S, 1991.

1991 Heart and Stroke Facts Statistics, American Heart Association, Dallas, Texas.

Index

sunflower seeds 61, 77, 128, 191
superoxide dismutase 244
sweating 242
sweet potatoes 20, 26, 129, 185

T-cells 25, 117
T'ai Chi 157
tang keui 53–4
tardive dyskinesia 132
taste loss 197–8
tea 30, 74–5
  chamomile 194
  club moss 45–7, 191–2
  herbal 175
  see also green tea
Teeguarden, R. 120
teeth, strong 35
temper 167–8
terpenes 45, 124
testosterone 233–4
thiamin 95, 127–8; see also
  vitamin B₁
throats, sore 54, 108
thyroid, overactive 39
tingling in the extremities 48
tinnitus 68
tocopherol 128–33, 186 see also
  vitamin E
tomatoes 21, 87, 97, 123
toothaches 54
tretinoin 133–4
tumour growth 51
tuna 101, 121, 137
turmeric 134–5, 161, 171, 174,
  177
turnips 86

ulcers 23, 86
ultraviolet light 27
unbelliferous vegetables 135–6
urinary tract infections (UTI)
  50–1, 118–19, 206
urination, excess 20

uterine cancer 14
uva-ursi 206

vaccination 7
vaginal bleeding 71, 203
vaginal dryness 53, 205–6
vaginal yeast infections 12
valerian 195
varicose veins 34, 35, 180,
  198–9
vascular disease 29
vasoconstrictors 34
vegetable oils 129; see also
  specific types
vegetables 17, 18, 29, 31, 86,
  112, 128, 162, 164, 196
  cruciferous 51–2, 126
  green, leafy 17, 18, 28, 58,
    61, 88, 91, 116, 191, 225
  root 104
  unbelliferous 135–6
  yellow 17, 18
  see also specific vegetables
ventricular fibrillation 102
viropause 220
vision 28, 145
  problems 8
  see also eyes, cataracts,
    macular degeneration
vitamins 9, 162–3
  A 25–6, 133, 134, 224
  B₁ (thiamin) 127–8, 190–1
  B₂ 116–17, 186, 241–2
  B₆ 117, 186, 205, 224
  B₁₂ 47–50
  C 19–21, 29, 30, 44, 72, 111,
    112, 113, 117, 169, 179,
    186, 203, 211, 244
  D 31, 35, 36, 136–7, 165,
    179, 215–17
  E 53, 94, 121, 122, 128–33,
    168, 173, 180, 186, 199,
    203, 205, 242